Cheap Meat

Cheap Meat

FLAP FOOD NATIONS IN
THE PACIFIC ISLANDS

Deborah Gewertz and
Frederick Errington

UNIVERSITY OF CALIFORNIA PRESS
Berkeley   Los Angeles   London

University of California Press, one of the most distinguished
university presses in the United States, enriches lives around the world
by advancing scholarship in the humanities, social sciences, and
natural sciences. Its activities are supported by the UC Press Foundation and by philanthropic contributions from individuals and
institutions. For more information, visit www.ucpress.edu.

University of California Press
Berkeley and Los Angeles, California

University of California Press, Ltd.
London, England

Library of Congress Cataloging-in-Publication Data

Gewertz, Deborah B., 1948–.
    Cheap meat : flap food nations in the pacific islands / Deborah
Gewertz and Frederick Errington.
        p.   cm.
    Includes bibliographical references and index.
    ISBN 978-0-520-26092-4 (cloth : alk. paper)
    ISBN 978-0-520-26093-1 (pbk. : alk. paper)
    1. Nutritional anthropology—Pacific Islands.   2. Lamb meat
industry—Pacific Islands.   3. Mutton industry—Pacific Islands.
4. Animal gut industries—Pacific Islands.   5. Food habits—Pacific
Islands.   6. Pacific Islands—Foreign economic relations—Australia.
7. Pacific Islands—Foreign economic relations—New Zealand.
I. Errington, Frederick Karl.   II. Title.

GN635.P27G49   2010
394.1'20996.5—dc22   2009020580

Manufactured in the United States of America

19   18   17   16   15   14   13   12
10   9   8   7   6   5   4   3

This book is printed on Cascades Enviro 100, a 100% post consumer
waste, recycled, de-inked fiber. FSC recycled certified and processed
chlorine free. It is acid free, Ecologo certified, and manufactured by
BioGas energy.

Contents

Illustrations

Acknowledgments

Thanking people for helping us with a multisited project involving a controversial topic is tricky. We spoke to many people in New Zealand, Australia, Papua New Guinea, and Fiji. And, if complete, the list might include some who would not wish to be mentioned. What to do? We have decided to limit the list to those who provided us with sociability as well as succor during our research—and to those we are relatively sure would not mind being acknowledged. We hope we do not offend in either direction of mentioning or not mentioning. In regard to all, we want to emphasize how much we learned. We have tried to listen carefully, and we have tried to write fairly. We do, of course, take full responsibility for what we have written.

We send our special gratitude to: Karen Brison, Mark Busse, Fiona Carruthers, Sneh Chand, Ann Chowning, Don Claasen, Ken Cokanasiga, Bob DeBourwere, Graeme Cook, Jope Davetanivalu, David Ellis, Ross Finlayson, Andy Fox, Hamish and Stratton Giblin, Claudia Gross, Tim Harrison, Philip Harvey, Trevor Hattersley, Judith Huntsman, Joseph

Kambukwat, Alfred Kerenga, Richard Kidd, David Kitchener, Philip Komai, Andrew Macpherson, Dennis McClenaghan, Ann and Fergus McLean, Peter Manueli, Gray Mathias, Ben O'Brien, Susan Parkinson, Mike Petersen, Chris Ritchie, Wila Saweri, Jimaima Schultz, Simon Sia, Rod Slater, Nancy Sullivan, Sidney and Sharifa Suma, Kerry Tate, Janet Tyson, Brian and Leanne Umbers, John Upton, and Mark Warren.

In addition, we would also like to recognize those who helped us gain institutional affiliation. In New Zealand, we thank Dr. Crispin Shore of the Department of Social Anthropology at the University of Auckland, who appointed us as Visiting Scholars.

In Papua New Guinea, we thank Dr. Peter Siba of the Papua New Guinea Medical Research Institute, who affiliated us and made us welcome. In Fiji, we thank Dr. Elise Huffer of the Pacific Studies Program of the University of the South Pacific. She recommended us to colleagues in the Ministries of Health and Education who vetted and approved our proposal.

Also, there are those who commented on aspects of our manuscript or helped us in its preparation in other ways. In addition to those mentioned in the book and those who provided anonymous reviews, we send our appreciation to Andy Anderson, George Armelagos, Alan Babb, Niko Besnier, Melissa Caldwell, James Carrier, Don Claasen, David Ellis, Robert Foster, Elizabeth Garland, Alan Goodman, Tim Harrison, Donna Hart, Surya Kundu, Peter Manueli, Ann McLean—and especially to Ella Kusnetz. We also benefited from discussion after we presented talks based on our research at the École des Hautes Études en Sciences Sociales, Johannes Gutenberg Institute, the University of Otago, the annual meetings of the Association for Social Anthropology in Oceania, and Amherst College.

Our research was financed by the National Science Foundation, grants 051322221 and 0512994; the American Council of Learned Societies; and the H. Axel Schupf '57 Fund for Intellectual Life Amherst College. We are very grateful for the support.

Finally, as always, we thank our luck for the opening of an elevator door.

INTRODUCTION **What's Not on Our Plates**

Our story is about a fatty, cheap meat eaten by peoples in the Pacific Islands, who are among the most overweight in the world. Lamb or mutton flaps—sheep bellies—are often 50 percent fat. They move from First World pastures and pens in New Zealand and Australia, where white people rarely eat them, to Third World pots and plates in the Pacific Islands, where brown people frequently eat them—and in large amounts.[1] As fatty and cheap meat, they are a kind of food implicated in the global epidemic of eating-related "lifestyle" diseases: obesity, diabetes, and hypertension. Many also implicate them in structures of inequality. The sale of lamb and mutton flaps to seemingly remote Pacific Islanders, we argue, involves political, ethical, and health issues of importance to us all.

In effect, our story about lamb and mutton flaps is both similar to and different from other accounts about food that have been told recently.[2]

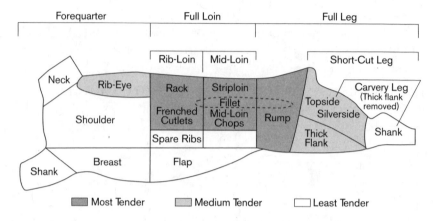

Figure 1. Lamb cuts

These tend to be of an "if you only knew" genre in their focus on how those in the First World are often ignorant of—indeed, often misled if not duped by—the corporate and industrial food system. In one variant, these accounts reveal that the foods we enjoy lack innocence by virtue of the circumstances of their production; in another, by virtue of their ingredients and environmental effects. Both—and they are often combined—are intended to provoke disquietude about injustice or ill-health (both personal and environmental) that might cause us to change our food choices or to protest in other ways.

The first variant, that revealing injustice, shows that the foods on our plates are often obtained at the expense of the foods not on other people's plates. Examples of this concern the tomatoes, green beans, broccoli, papayas, pineapples, and coffee produced for export by disadvantaged farmers and farm workers living in Mexico, Zambia, Guatemala, Jamaica, Mexico, the Philippines, and Papua New Guinea.[3] Other examples concern the domestically produced chickens, pigs, cows, and fruit that are often plucked, slaughtered, or picked by undocumented immigrants from poorer countries living uneasily among us.[4] These accounts—about what it takes to get us what we eat—make for sobering tales of the tactics of transnational food corporations.[5] Demonstrating as they do the exploitation of the lives of others, they shake up our complacency.[6]

The second variant, that revealing ill health, shows that what is in the food on our plates is often not good for us or for our planet. A particularly engaging example of this sort is Michael Pollan's *The Omnivore's Dilemma*.[7] The dilemma is that, as omnivores living in contemporary contexts, many people must choose from a wide array of palatable foods, some of which may prove deleterious. Pollan shows, for instance, how much of the food easily available to us is the product of an industrial, corn-based food chain running from fields to feedlots, factories, and supermarkets. This industrial food chain provides us with nutritionally dubious foods formulated to maximize appeal through reliance on fat and sweets.[8] It also relies on environmentally dubious practices formulated to maximize yield with the help of pesticides, herbicides, fertilizers, hormones, and antibiotics. Pollan and others provide sobering discussions of the physiological and environmental effects of transnational food corporations in their hunger for profit. In demonstrating the exploitation of our health and our environment, they too shake up our complacency.

There are, of course, Pacific Island examples that could lend themselves to the "if you only knew" renditions of both variants. Many of these are known not only to us, but also to a range of activists and health professionals, both from the Pacific Islands and elsewhere, who have written about the deplorable conditions under which many Pacific Islanders labor to produce foods for export to First World countries and the adverse environmental effects of this industry. An especially egregious case is that of RD Tuna in Papua New Guinea, which, under the guise of providing much-needed development, pays workers badly, strips the local seas clean of tuna and other fish, and dumps factory effluent.[9] And many Pacific Islanders eat energy-dense industrial foods that are globally ubiquitous. These include the likes of Twisties, which are made and distributed throughout the Pacific and eaten not only as a snack but often as a meal. Made by PepsiCo., Twisties are a corn and rice preparation (resembling Cheetos, the product familiar to U.S. snackers) that is extruded into hot vegetable oil and then artificially colored and flavored to form salty, greasy, crunchy, cheese- or chicken-favored, spiral-shaped bites. Also popular with Pacific Islanders are the instant noodles such as

Nestle's Maggi,[10] which contain wheat flour, vegetable oil, salt, wheat gluten, mineral salts, vegetable gum, and artificial colors; the flavor mix that accompanies them is extremely salty and contains artificial flavor enhancers (specifically, monosodium glutamate and disodium 5 ribonucleotide), anticaking agents (specifically, sodium aluminum silicate and calcium phosphates), hydrolysed plant protein, maltodextrin, onion powder, vegetable fats, parsley flakes, and flavor extracts.

Our story about lamb and mutton flaps as they move from New Zealand and Australia to the Pacific Islands can also be placed in this "if you only knew" genre. We reveal things about cheap, fatty meat that our readers probably do not know. And, like other accounts in this genre, ours does convey a politics. However, there are some important and instructive differences between our story and those of the others we have mentioned. First of all, flaps are not brought to anyone's plates—whether First or Third World—under shockingly oppressive labor conditions. They are produced and processed in New Zealand and Australia under relatively reasonable and regulated work circumstances. Neither are they brought to anyone's plates under biologically and environmentally deleterious circumstances. They are an unadulterated cut from grass-fed sheep. Flaps, in other words, do not hide dirty little secrets of either origin or ontology. They are simply very fatty meat.

Yet, as fatty meat par excellence, their trade to the Pacific Islands is politically charged: too fatty to be eaten by the (mostly) white people who produce and purvey them, they go out to a region that includes the seven countries with the world's highest percentage of overweight adults.[11] Our story, therefore, is about an instructive and salient extreme: a First to Third World trade that brings the epitome of fatty meat to those with the epitome of fatty bodies.[12] Given all of the foods that Pacific Islanders do eat—including the industrial foods just mentioned—we do not claim that lamb and mutton flaps are the central causes of obesity or other forms of ill health there. In fact, from what we have learned, it is not necessarily the case that eating fatty meat contributes significantly more to lifestyle diseases than eating the equivalent calories in refined starches and sugars. (As Dr. Walter Willett, an epidemiologist at Harvard University and Chair of the Department of Nutrition, explained to us in an e-mail communication, "Reducing sheep fat [in the diets of Pacific Islanders] would probably not have much benefit unless replaced with a polyunsaturated oil or overall fewer calories. Reducing refined starches and sugar would have more benefit.")[13] However, because the analogies suggested by flaps are so clear and vivid—fatty (sheep) flesh makes fatty (Pacific Island) bodies—they become convenient and compelling symbols of what many people see as unequal relationships between whole categories of differently located people—some eating and others eschewing, some becoming rich and others becoming sick. In addition, whereas a small Pacific Island government is unlikely to make the argument that all products containing, for instance, disodium 5 ribonucleotide or sodium silicate must be tariffed or banned, the obvious fattiness of flaps has made them a convenient and compelling focus for national political attention.[14] For those in the Pacific Islands, flaps both stand for and contribute to a regional variant of the omnivore's dilemma: that of being able to make the right food choices. This is to say, the story we tell is somewhat unlike the others of the genre because we are interested not in compelling a politics, but in exploring one that already is flourishing. Following the flaps involves not only tracing a commodity, but also probing a controversy.

FLIP-FLAPPING THROUGH THE PACIFIC

In tracing this commodity and probing this controversy, we build upon our own history as anthropologists, especially in the country of Papua New Guinea. First arriving when Papua New Guinea was still, in effect, a colony of Australia (in the late 1960s, for Fred, and early 1970s, for Deborah), we have made many subsequent field trips over the past thirty years. These field trips led to projects about a range of subjects, many of them focused on change: traditional ritual as well as evangelical Christianity; clan organization as well as class formation; male initiation through skin cutting as well as university graduation through test taking; fish for sago barter markets as well as canned mackerel and rice-purveying trade stores. To make sense of how lives were changing, we focused on such broad processes of modernity as the frequent movement of Papua

New Guineans from their subsistence-rich villages to impoverished urban settlements.[15] We attempted to understand how and why they came
to find urban life desirable despite its only marginal feasibility—despite
(as we have personally observed in squatter settlements) malnutrition, if
not chronic hunger. In this regard, we became interested specifically in
changing food systems and how they came to feature in the stories people
told about what life should offer. For instance, members of the new urban
elite often told us that they would never return to their home villages
where there was no assured access to "the little bags of sugar" to which
they had become accustomed. Or they told us—sometimes boasting,
sometimes lamenting—that their children insisted on store-bought food
when visiting their grandparents back in the village. In addition, our less
affluent urban friends told us, as a demonstration of their capacity for sophisticated coping, which trade-store had the best prices on which urban
staples such as rice, canned fish, and sugar. They also appraised the quality of their squatter settlement life—both its transformed modernity and
its persisting traditionality—in terms of the opportunities it offered for
relaxing and sharing a beer or a Coke with kinsmen.

Related to our interest in change, we for some time taught classes about
the anthropology of food. In one such course we showed a film, aptly
entitled *Hungry for Profit*, which describes the effects of "agribusiness"
on much of the Third World.[16] In its castigation of many multinational
corporations for their Third World depredations, one company, Booker
Tate Limited, was exempted. We subsequently discovered that Booker
Tate had developed and now managed Papua New Guinea's only sugar
plantation, Ramu Sugar Limited (RSL), which provided the "little bags"
of such significance to many of our Papua New Guinean friends. Our
interests multiply converging and piqued, we asked and were given permission to write a historically informed ethnography exploring how RSL
had come into being, how it worked, and where it was going.[17]

It was during our initial visit to RSL in 1999 that we first became
aware of lamb and mutton flaps. (In retrospect, we realized that the di-
lapidated urban dwelling where we lived in 1994 was probably patched
with cartons once containing lamb and mutton flaps that had been called
into service as building material because of their weather-resistant,

waxed linings.) We soon learned that for many Papua New Guineans at RSL, eating cheap fatty meat in the form of imported flaps was central to a modernist good life, a life which met at least some of their aspirations. Thus, whenever we asked what we could bring to church functions or other communal gatherings, we were usually told to bring frozen flaps, which were readily available at one of the local mini-supermarkets. And every payday we would find the supermarket freezers surrounded by eager customers sorting through the packages of flaps to find those with the optimal balance of bones, fat, and flesh to make a savory and afford-able meal when mixed with local greens, rice, or other carbohydrates. Why had we never heard of flaps before we worked at RSL? What, we began to wonder, brought such meat to our Papua New Guinea friends? And how had it become so central in their lives—at least to their ideas of what their lives should be like?

In effect, our RSL project was an attempt to understand processes of globalization as they have come together in one place. We had to con-sider, among other topics, the agro-industrial practices of growing sugar-cane, the elaborate technology of sugar processing, the contingencies of trade, tariffs, and financing. We had to understand the desires of Papua New Guinean nationalists who wanted for their new nation (indepen-dent from Australia in 1975) not only a sugar industry, but one located in a single, agro-industrial complex. We had to explore the perspectives of RSL's Papua New Guinean employees, who were drawn from many of the country's almost eight hundred linguistic groups. We had to investi-gate the reasons why nearby villagers chose to give up subsistence agri-culture to grow sugarcane for the company. We had to probe the lives of the expatriate Britons for whom RSL was one assignment in a career of international sugar advising. And we had to learn how all these forces and kinds of people worked together (or not). It was our endeavor—one central to anthropology—to see material forces and processes in histori-cally and culturally located contexts of meaning and purpose.

To do all of this, we used many of the methodologies familiar to "tradi-tional" anthropologists—specifically those that produce the detailed, nuanced, and context-sensitive observations that constitute what has been called "thick description."[18] We settled down for a substantial period of time and engaged in "participant observation": trying to learn what was happening by immersing ourselves in the daily lives of those directly affected by RSL. And, as anthropologists have long done, we supplemented this immersion with formal interviews and archival research. Yet if our RSL project was a place-centered study of globalism—a study of convergence—our present project is a multisited study of globalism—a study of divergence. As we have said, flaps are produced and processed in New Zealand and Australia and then fan outward as exports to the Pacific Islands and elsewhere. Although place no longer organizes this new study, our objectives remain much as they were, as do many of our techniques. We still work to see material forces and processes as historically located and culturally inflected. And we still use the techniques of participant observation, formal interviews, and archival research.

To follow the flow of flaps and to understand the controversy about them has demanded, in addition, a somewhat novel strategy—a multisited approach. No longer focused on gaining an intimate knowledge of a place and those centered there, this strategy runs the risk of sacrificing the local to the global, the deep for the broad, the thick for the thin.[19] One way of overcoming the problem is to station several anthropologists along the network through which a commodity moves. Another, more anthropologically popular, technique—and the one that we chose, partly because supporting a team of investigators is a difficult proposition—is to build on the researcher's own field experience in a part of the world where the commodity originates, passes through, or is consumed.

However, while we could build on our anthropological knowledge about Papua New Guinea, we did have to establish ourselves as fieldworkers in places we had previously only visited as tourists. Thus for three months in 2004 and five months in 2006 we interviewed as many New Zealanders as we could who had an interest in, or at least knowledge about, the commerce in lamb and mutton flaps: the traders, processors, and farmers of the meat industry; the specialists in trade and Pacific affairs of the government; the physicians and epidemiologists of the public health sector. Then we traveled to Australia and spent several weeks interviewing meat traders and public health specialists who focus on the Pacific Islands.

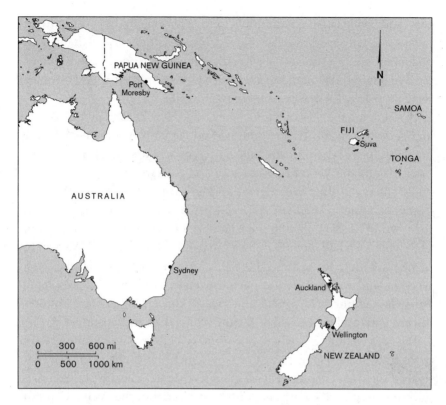

Figure 2.   The Pacific islands of most importance for our project

We chose to do substantially more research in New Zealand than in Australia for several reasons. New Zealand is the world's largest exporter of sheep meat (supplying about 75 percent of the world export market) and dominates much of the Pacific Island market. Even in Papua New Guinea, still strongly tied to Australia by virtue of geography and postcolonial politics, New Zealand commands a substantial share of the lamb and mutton flap trade. Moreover, for the purpose of studying the complexities of the Pacific Island–centered meat trade as thickly as possible, a greater focus on New Zealand had clear advantages. New Zealand is of more manageable scale, both in terms of geography and population, than Australia. Visits to all parts of the country are relatively easy, and contacts quickly multiply, since everyone in the meat industry knows virtually everyone else. Indeed, New Zealanders joke that it takes no more than three phone calls to link you with anyone else in the country. We should also mention that we have well-placed friends in New Zealand who helped us with these phone calls.

In following the flow of flaps as they leave New Zealand and Australia and enter the Pacific, we concentrated on Papua New Guinea, which is not only a place where we had much prior experience but also the largest Pacific Island market for flaps. In 2004 and 2006 we interviewed import-ers, retailers, health professionals, and government representatives. We examined issues related to flaps in particular and diet more generally in the town of Madang among the Chambri, members of a cultural group with whom we had already done a great deal of fieldwork.[20] We also re-turned to RSL to learn more about the "shopping baskets" of plantation workers, and we arranged to have university students visit five Papua New Guinea towns to conduct interviews concerning general attitudes toward flaps and the occasions during which they are consumed.[21]

We next went to Fiji, where our primary objective was to understand more fully the reasons and means by which the country, in 2000, had banned the sale of flaps. In Fiji we interviewed public health professionals, government officials, members of the Secretariat of the Pacific Commu-nity, and meat importers. We also arranged to have two graduate students conduct 185 interviews, again concerning the occasions when people had eaten flaps and their attitudes toward them, and in this case whether they thought the ban was necessary and successful. Our study also included library research on the Pacific Island of Tonga and interviews with health professionals active there, even though we were not able to travel to the island. Tonga has an exceptionally serious problem with lifestyle diseases, and the government is currently struggling to regulate the import of all fatty meats, especially of lamb and mutton flaps.

Our project has been to understand and bring together the range of perspectives of those linked, directly or indirectly, in this contentious trade.[22] This presents us with an anthropological challenge and a hope. The challenge is to write with the assumption that what we say will not simply be sequestered in the academy, but will also be read by those whose perspectives we are representing. We must accept that we are accountable to what are, in effect, multiple constituencies. Multisited research, thus, implies multisited responsibilities to get the story right, or at least relatively so: to thicken the often thin understandings that various constituencies have of one another, and to thicken such understandings so that all concerned may come to appreciate more fully the contexts in which they and the others live.[23] Yet in addressing issues of political contention—after engaging with all of the various constituencies that participate in the trade in flaps—we must also accept an obligation to struggle toward a position that conveys a policy.

ONE Thinking about Meat

During one of the first conversations we had with a New Zealand meat trader about the politically controversial sale of lamb and mutton flaps from his country and Australia to the Pacific Islands, he stopped to make sure we understood something very basic about his enterprise and the market: You do realize, he said, that no one grows a sheep for its flaps; the reason flaps don't bring a very good price is because they are too fatty for people who can afford better. But we will be able to sell them some-place when the price gets right. Meat never goes uneaten. It's that simple.

We had not thought about flaps in quite such succinct terms before, but we certainly understood what he was saying. In fact, we had become interested in flaps partly because they are usually avoided by white New Zealanders and Australians yet eagerly sought by many Pacific Islanders. For the former, flaps, which contain less than 50 percent lean meat, are visibly too fatty to seem appealing or healthful. For the latter, flaps are too cheap and plentiful to be passed over. Indeed, the less affluent countries of the nearby Pacific Islands are a ready market for the export from New Zealand and Australia of large volumes of these low-value cuts (though 9–12 percent of a sheep's carcass by weight, flaps are only 3–5 percent of its value). Thus, while peripheral to the centrally located trader, flaps are central to our friends on the periphery. Of course, as the meat trader knows, however simple marketing principles of supply and demand may be, actually trading flaps, especially into the Pacific Islands, is rarely simple. Such trade involves more than grasping the global opportunity of turning one people's trash into another's treasure. Because, as we shall see, those who treasure flaps know that they are rejected as trash by those who provide them, this trade is, at the least, politically sensitive.[1] But such complexities temporarily aside, the meat traders do seem to be correct in a fundamental recognition: meat never goes uneaten. And this seems to have been the case for a very long time.

HUMANS AS MEAT EATERS

No one can be certain about the significance of meat eating to our earliest ancestors. Scholars speculate and infer based upon incomplete evidence in their attempts to reconstruct when, where, and why those who evolved into *Homo sapiens* began to eat meat with regularity. They also speculate and infer concerning the physiological and cultural effects of meat eating in human evolution. However, we are not anthropologists who specialize in reconstructing this evolution. All we can do is briefly convey what makes sense to us given what we have read.

In considering the role of meat in the lives of our ancestors, we think it important to avoid some of the assumptions about gender and human nature that are associated with the classic "man the hunter" argument. This argument has been rightly criticized as discounting the role of women and their gathering in human evolution. In fact, female gathering likely provided the calories that could be relied on for daily survival.[2] In addition, the argument has been rightly criticized as fostering the stereotype of humans—men in particular—as fundamentally violent.[3] In fact, male hunting likely provided important contexts for trust and social solidarity through cooperation and food sharing.

This being said, there is widespread—though not universal—agreement that our earliest ancestors ate meat whenever possible.[4] They could, it seems, digest meat with relative ease. Initially, raw meat acquired through scavenging and opportunistic hunting was a nutritionally dense supplement to the raw roots and tubers available in the woodlands of Africa.[5] As human evolution continued, meat remained an important component of the diet. And, at some point (perhaps as early as two million years ago[6]), our ancestors began to cook. While cooking enabled a wider range of plant foods (including those otherwise toxic) to be exploited, its greatest value was in helping our ancestors to extract more nutrients, more easily, from all of their foods—plant as well as animal.[7] With increased nutrition, stature increased. In addition, with the availability of plant and animal foods that were easily chewed and readily digested, both tooth size and gut size decreased. Hence, the nutritional benefits of meat eating and cooking may have been important in the gradual (400,000-year) transition from the short-statured, large-toothed, big-gutted, small-brained members of the genus *Australopithecus* into the taller, smaller, slimmer, and larger variants of the genus *Homo*.[8]

The decrease in gut size was itself perhaps significant because it, in turn, may have facilitated an increase in brain size. Brains are expensive tissues to provision. Evidence of this comes from physical anthropologist William Leonard. He reports that a contemporary adult human (at rest) uses 20–25 percent of his or her energy needs to maintain brain metabolism, while nonhuman primates use 8–10 percent.[9] Such facts have been interpreted by some to suggest that large human brains could not have been adequately sustained under early gathering and hunting circumstances without the reduction of another major metabolic system. There might, in other words, have been insufficient calories to support both a big brain and a big gut.[10] Others are content to argue that a better diet resulting from an increase in meat eating (and eventually by cooking) was enough to foster the development of the human brain. Largely in support of the latter perspective, Leonard writes, "For early *Homo*, acquiring more gray matter meant seeking out more of the energy-dense fare"—namely, animal foods.[11]

At a certain point, increased brain size and the development of culture proved mutually reinforcing. Simply put, smarter people with more sophisticated ways of organizing, innovating, and interpreting their surroundings became more successful as they encountered one another and expanded through diverse environments. Culture, once elaborated, became *Homo*'s master adaptation. In its elaboration—in the development of ways of organizing, innovating, and interpreting—meat eating continued to have a role.[12] Cooking allowed nutrients to be better extracted from the relatively reliable vegetable food base (again, confirming the importance of woman in gathering) so that more time and energy could be spent over greater distances in hunting for nutritionally dense meats (which could, in addition, be preserved through smoking). Success in hunting, in turn, both relied on and further encouraged the development of the broadly adaptive strategies of cooperation and food sharing. Hence the increased emphasis on hunting that was facilitated by cooking may itself have contributed, at least in a small way, to the transition to a smarter and more culture-dependent *Homo*.

Significantly, as hunting techniques and technologies improved and as hominids spread out of Africa, large herbivores (including very large ones, such as mammoths) became prized game.[13] In fact, Leonard believes that early humans may have spread widely out of Africa initially in pursuit of migrating animal herds.[14] According to the geographer and environmental ecologist Vaclav Smil, such large herbivores would certainly have been more desirable than monkeys, hares, rabbits, and small deer—animals that might yield only two to three times the amount of energy expended in killing them. Large herbivores, with their larger body mass and (often) greater fat, might have more than twice the energy density of these smaller species.[15] To be sure, they were big and often dangerous, but the payoff from a successful hunt would be great. According to Smil, if a group was lucky enough to kill a mammoth, its members would have access to between thirty and fifty times as much energy as the energy that had been expended in making the kill.[16] On the other hand, physical anthropologists John Speth and Katherine

Spielmann argue that, at particular seasons, such large herbivores as bison and caribou may have been seriously fat-depleted and therefore less desirable energy sources than some smaller species. For instance, beaver and bear—and some fish—were likely to be relatively fat even in the later winter and early spring. Nonetheless, all agree that protein from meat sources was both necessary and valued.[17] (We return to the significance of *fatty* animal protein a bit later.)

Some ten thousand years ago, however, such hunting and gathering subsistence strategies became less viable in certain areas of the world such as the Middle East, where agriculture became both feasible and necessary. Although agriculture did allow for larger population densities, it also led to a decline in the amount of meat—fatty or not—available for most people. Smil estimates that "average per capita meat intakes in traditional agricultural societies were rarely higher than 5–10 kg a year," while preagricultural intakes were no less than 6–17 kg per year and, in many environments, 10–20 kg per year.[18] Concerning peasant societies in the Old World, he writes that "meat was eaten no more frequently than once a week and relatively large amounts were consumed, as roasts and stews, only during festive occasions. . . . Consequently, animal foods provided generally less than 15 percent of all dietary protein, and saturated animal fats supplied just around 10 percent of all food energy in preindustrial populations."[19] In fact, until relatively recently in the Old World, meat was reserved mostly for ruling elites, wealthy urbanites, and marching armies; most people seldom ate meat.

Meat's value thus derives from a complex of reasons. It is energy-dense and, when limited in availability, is often associated with wealth and privilege. It is, in addition, a food suggestive of existential and moral considerations. Because its acquisition involves the death of creatures that are clearly analogous to humans, it often carries with it considerations of life, death, and reproduction as well as those of reciprocity between species, spirits, and social groups.[20] For example, among the horticultural, though forest-dwelling, Kaluli of Papua New Guinea, men would hunt for weeks to amass the smoked meat necessary for the ceremonial exchanges that linked kin and neighbors throughout a particular region in relationships of positive reciprocity. At the same time,

Kaluli cosmology posits animals—especially wild pigs—and humans as linked in reciprocity. The world of one is the mirror of the other: humans in the Kaluli world appear as wild pigs to those in the other world, and vice versa. Hence Kaluli pig hunts result in the deaths of humans in the other world, and Kaluli deaths are often attributed to pig hunts by the mirrored others.[21] A comparable cosmology is found among the horticultural Wari of the South American Amazon. There people become white-lipped peccaries when they die and are believed to offer themselves up to living kinsmen as game.[22]

As a final example, and one closer to home, the anthropologist Nick Fiddes argues that it is precisely in the Old World—influenced as it eventually became by the Judeo-Christian tradition—that meat became an apt expression of God's relationship to man. According to the Bible, God gives man "dominion over the fish of the sea, and over the fowl of the air, and over the cattle, and over all the earth, and over every creeping thing that creepeth upon the earth."[23] Under these circumstances, meat becomes, in Fiddes's phrase, a "natural symbol": one that is tangible and easy to understand and comes "naturally" to hand as a way to represent human control of the natural world. Indeed, he says, "Consuming the muscle flesh of other highly evolved animals is a potent statement of our supreme power."[24] Such power—the power to kill sentient animals for one's own benefit—can be not only gratifying in its assertion of human pre-eminence, but also discomfiting, as shown by efforts to distinguish the "animal from the edible"—for instance, in calling the living creature a *cow* and its flesh, *beef*.[25]

Energy-dense, difficult to acquire, and socially and symbolically meaningful, meat does seem to be special. Even for those relatively few who actively refuse meat—who, for instance, strongly object to the assertion of human preeminence—it can be argued that meat remains salient if only as "that which must be rejected." And when people gain increased access to such a multifaceted good, they usually eat more of it. By the nineteenth century, especially in Western Europe and the United States, industrialization, urbanization, and greater agricultural productivity that allowed livestock to be fed grains began to provide such access. As Friedrich Engels noted in 1844 in *Condition of the Working-Class in England,* "The better-paid workers, especially those in whose families every member is able to earn something, have good food as long as this state of things lasts; meat daily, and bacon and cheese for supper. Where wages are less, meat is used only two or three times a week, and the proportion of bread and potatoes increases. Descending gradually, we find the animal food reduced to a small piece of bacon cut up with the potatoes; lower still, even this disappears."[26]

Meat consumption would continue to increase in Europe, although, as the statement from Engels suggests, the rich were likely to eat more of it than the poor. If one extrapolates from aggregate figures of carcass weight provided by Smil, it appears that the amount of meat eaten by the British tripled during the nineteenth century to a per capita consumption of 40 kg a year by 1900; the amount eaten by the French remained stable through the first half of the nineteenth century and then doubled over the next eighty years to more than 35 kg; and the amount consumed by Americans reached 51 kg by 1909.[27] In fact, as early as 1851 a working-class family in New York would buy annually about 66 kg of fresh meat per person (at about ten cents per pound). To be sure, these would be cheaper cuts for stewing and boiling, bones for soup stock, and an occasional roast or steak purchased for special occasions.[28]

These trends in increased meat consumption have continued, and not just among those in the industrialized world. With increasingly globalized food systems, says Jeffery Sobal, "the dietary and nutritional transitions from plant-based high-fiber diets to animal- and vegetable-oil based, low-fiber, high-fat, high-protein diets" is spreading "to an increasing proportion of the world's population."[29] According to statistics collected by the Food and Agricultural Organization during 2000, those in affluent countries worldwide consumed a mean of 53 kg/year of meat, and in modernizing ones, 18 kg/year (although there is controversy over this figure because China seems to have inflated its statistics; see below).[30] Adam Drewnowski, an epidemiologist, supplies supplementary and more finely grained statistics, estimating that in Japan the per capita consumption of beef, veal, pork, and poultry rose from 2.2 kg in 1955 to 30 kg in 1994, while in China the consumption of these meats rose from 8 kg in 1970 to 35.8 in 1994.[31]

Indeed, for many poorer people meat has become the marker of modernity, a topic we explore in some detail later in this book. Thus the anthropologist Sarah Mahler found that among Central and South American migrants to the United States, increased access to meat is one of the few satisfactory aspects of their experience.[32] Though the lives to which they aspire often remain out of reach—the nice cars they lean against in the pictures they send home are not theirs—they do feel affluent in terms of what they can eat. According to the historian Roger Horowitz, "When the relatively marginal gained more buying power, their meat consumption grew dramatically. . . . Meat is coveted and immigrants can be seen in the supermarket aisles pushing shopping carts laden heavily with packages of beef and chicken."[33] Certainly the link between meat and modernity is clear to those enjoying the cheap and fatty lamb and mutton flaps in the Pacific Islands.

ON FATTY MEAT IN PARTICULAR

Human beings thus have long liked meat. But the trader with whom we began was not only saying that meat, by virtue of its universal appeal, will always find a market. He was also saying that some cuts of meat will find a market more readily than others. Even lamb and mutton flaps, deemed too fatty for some, will find a home if they are priced right. What do we make, then, of the fact that very fatty meats are likely to be of low value in terms of desirability and price?

Humans do tend to appreciate at least some fat on their meat. Large herbivores, as we have mentioned, were particularly sought after as food by stone-age hunters not only because they were large but also because they were fatty (though not as fatty as contemporary domesticated animals).[34] The anthropologist Marvin Harris goes so far as to suggest that much of the craving for meat is actually a craving for fatty meat. Fat is essential for the processing of the fat-soluble vitamins necessary for human health. Fat is also particularly useful because it is energy-dense and can be used readily to fuel the body. Unless there is such an energy source present in the diet, the amino acids in meat will be diverted, becoming fuel rather than body-building proteins. Correspondingly, "hunters run the risk of starving to death if they rely too much on lean meat."[35]

Fat is also appreciated because many people find that fatty meats smell good when cooked. Though much of meat is composed of water, its aroma-carrying molecules are "hydrophobic" and can be dissolved in and conveyed by the fat alone. Therefore fat contributes significantly to the savory smell of cooking/cooked meat.[36] And if it is true, as some have suggested, that humans possess taste receptors for fat, then smell and taste would complement each other.[37] Indeed, it could be argued that fat became useful in human evolution for both its smell and its taste, which alert humans not just to high-energy foods, but also to protein-rich foods that could be used for their body-building amino acids.[38]

Finally, fat is appreciated because it contributes to tenderness in three ways. According to Harold McGee in his magisterial *On Food and Cooking*, "Fat cells interrupt and weaken the sheet of connective tissue and the mass of muscle fibers; fat melts when heated rather than drying out and stiffening as the fibers do; and it lubricates the tissue, helping to separate fiber from fiber. Without much fat, otherwise tender meat becomes compacted, dry, and tough."[39]

Thus, as Horowitz shows in his study of meat in the U.S. diet, in the mid-1800s in New York City, roasts and steaks cut from the loin and rib were considered the most desirable, while "tougher cuts, such as the flank, rounds (both from the hind quarters), brisket, and plate (the latter two from the forequarters), generally served for stews, as longer cooking times in water soften them sufficiently. Bony meat, such as the neck, shoulder, and thigh, was 'excellent for a sweet, strengthening soup.' . . . Poor residents could even obtain beef shins, though they were 'fit for nothing but soup.'"[40] Least desirable, however, were the fatty trimmings removed from more valuable cuts as well as the offal. Much of this leftover material, from both cows and pigs, was (and still is) combined with meat and other ingredients and disguised in sausages. Here, for example, are New York recipes popular at the turn of the twentieth century for frankfurters. One used seventy pounds of shoulder trimmings, twenty pounds of knuckle meat and about sixty pounds from the pig's fat back to form a mixture about 40 percent fat—to which water, seasoning, and preservatives were added. Another recipe called for about sixty-five pounds of cheek meat, fifteen pounds of tripe, twenty-five pounds of kidneys, and seventy-seven pounds of regular pork trimmings—which were mostly fat and rind. Corn meal, accounting for about 10 percent of the frankfurters' weight, was then added so as to "help conceal high fat content by retarding shrinkage during cooking."[41]

What constitutes *excessive* fat content is, of course, at least partly determined by context. This context is a product not only of what else one is eating but also of shifting standards of beauty, health, and well-being. As numerous sources have documented, what constitutes an appropriate level of visible fat in meats has changed for many in Western countries, including those white New Zealanders and Australians for whom lamb and mutton flaps are just too obviously fatty to be acceptable even as cheap meat.[42] Yet, as many of us know, serious efforts to cut down on fat consumption may be difficult, especially when fat is concealed—tasted but not seen.[43] Indeed, there is some evidence that eating fat may become addictive—that fatty meat may not only be good to eat, but good to keep on eating.[44] And, to anticipate a bit, when fats are linked to sugars, as they increasingly are in fast foods, the combination may be both insidious and irresistible. Added to the human enjoyment of fats is an apparently innate human fondness for sugars. The results are the perfect, nutritionally dubious snacks which, as Sidney Mintz said, are both crisp and "finger-licking good."[45]

MORE ON MOVING FATTY MEAT INTO FATTY BODIES

We now have a better and more detailed understanding of what the trader told us about the fundamental nature of his business: Because humans like meat, often with some measure of fat, meat never goes uneaten (and it may, in fact, be overeaten). Although there is likely to be a hierarchy among cuts of meat, traders will be able to sell virtually all of these cuts somewhere, if the price is right. And the mechanisms of the market work effectively to convey cuts that are more or less expensive by virtue of their desirability to those who can afford them. However, the trader also recognized that there were special complexities (unfortunate ones, he thought) in the Pacific Island trade in lamb and mutton flaps, and it was, after all, these complexities that had brought us to him.

During the course of our research, we spoke to many white New Zealanders and Australians about our interest in flaps. Most had never eaten them. Some told us that they used to eat them when they were growing up in rural areas, but more frequently they had fed them to their dogs. Such a practice has remained common among sheep farmers; a recent article in *New Zealand Farmers Weekly* recommended that even if flaps are not available from sheep killed on the farm, they should still be acquired and fed to working dogs once or twice a week.[46] Others we talked to said that they ate flaps during their impoverished student days because they were cheap. But even for this minority, consumption of flaps was something they had left behind. Interestingly, the fact that flaps are no longer viewed as appropriate fare stimulated one New Zealand man's efforts to redeem them. He was prompted by the recollection that "when he was a kid, his father would buy and butcher half a lamb at a time so that he could get cheap meat and tasty lamb flaps featured regularly." In his article "Barbecue Lamb Belly the Slow Way" (interestingly subtitled "Or How I Wasted My Saturday Afternoon"), he describes how, after trimming the flaps and giving the scraps to his cat, he grilled them for four hours with the idea that "if lamb flap is slow-cooked, most of the fat will render out." Along the way he mentions that flaps are "as good as currency in New Guinea."[47]

We should mention as well that some seek out fatty meats precisely because they are not generally seen as appropriate fare. The *New York Times* writer Frank Bruni describes some upscale New York restaurants as catering to such transgressive eating. Bruni believes that "decades of proliferating sushi and shrinking plates, of clean California cuisine and exhortations to graze, have fostered a robust (or is that rotund?) counterculture of chefs and diners eager to cut against the nutritional grain and straight into the bellies of beasts. In fact, bellies (most often pork, more recently lamb) are this counterculture's LSD."[48] Said one restaurant patron, eating such food "puts you in touch with your barbaric self."

However, transgressors aside, the fact that most white New Zealanders and Australians (not to mention Americans) do not desire lamb and mutton flaps and Papua New Guineans and other Pacific Islanders do reflects more than a distribution of preferences and incomes. It seems to reflect a real dichotomy between those who produce but eschew the product and those who import and enjoy it: between those for whom flaps are not good enough and those for whom flaps are just fine. And this dichotomy suggests not only differences in who can afford to buy what, but also in who is better than whom. Thus the trade in flaps, at least in the Pacific Islands, is not a simple matter of supply and demand. Rather, it is a complex and political matter filled with connotations about comparability and worth. Moreover, because this is a trade in fatty flesh, the complexities often become embodied in fatty Pacific Island flesh in a manner that compels attention and demands response.

As we have suggested, the prevalence of eating-related lifestyle—also known as "non-communicable"—diseases among many Pacific Islanders is alarming.[49] In Tonga, the obesity prevalence among those aged fifteen and above is more than 60 percent; 29 percent of Tongans die of cardiovascular diseases, the leading causes of death for them. The rate of diabetes is also very high; at about 15 percent of the population (having doubled in prevalence from 7.5 percent in 1973 to 15.1 percent in 2002), Tonga's prevalence of diabetes and impaired glucose tolerance is among the highest in the world.[50]

Although a genetic component is likely in such high rates of lifestyle diseases,[51] it is also clear that some Tongans are eating too much and not very well. As one dramatic illustration, a Japanese journalist described the usual pre-diet daily fare of an affluent Tongan woman, 5 feet 8 inches tall, who at one point weighed 290 pounds before a successful effort at weight reduction:[52]

Breakfast: 6 fried eggs, 5 pieces of bread, 110 g of butter, plenty of jam or preserves, plenty of sugar, and any leftovers from the previous night.

Lunch: 1 kg. of *sipi* [the local term for flaps], 8 ripe bananas, 1 kg. of root crops.

Dinner: Same as lunch.

Snacks: 1 liter of ice-cream, or 6 pancakes, or half a cake.

This woman did decide to cut back, but what should be done, not only for her but for Tongans more generally? A study carried out by the South Pacific Consumer Protection Programme, requested by Tonga's National Food and Nutrition Committee as part of its efforts to confront the country's lifestyle diseases, recognized that "Consumers do have a choice. Everyday we choose what food we prepare for our family. If we choose to prepare a regular diet of fatty foods (like mutton flaps), our families' health will be at risk; if we choose a diet of fresh local food our family will be healthier. The problem is that Pacific Island peoples have a limited choice in the market place because we have limited cash to buy food and because traders persist in importing, and offering for sale, poor quality cuts of meat like mutton flaps."[53] In other words, though choice is important, it is also shaped and constrained. As the report concluded, the presence of flaps in the Pacific Islands is controversial—and "the answer [about what to do concerning them] is not that simple."

SOME MEATY IDEAS

Because the answer is not simple—because flaps are fatty meat, desired by some, though not by those who produce and purvey them, and because they become part of fatty bodies—they are a commodity worth anthropological attention. They have effects and are understood by differently located people to have effects in a regional (if not world) system. This is a system in which First World nations are complexly and often ambiguously linked to Third World nations. Certainly, throughout the region, these differently located people pay considerable attention to where flaps come from, where they go, and with what apparent consequences in wealth and in health. Flaps, thus observed, become caught up in the ways in which these people identify themselves and others. The fact that some eat flaps and others avoid them is recognized not just as a reflection of personal preference (as, perhaps, with eating or avoiding broccoli) but as a mark of group membership. Simply put, flap eaters are seen as distinguished in important ways from flap refusers. In this regard, flaps operate much as do "totems."

As anthropologists use the term, *totems* are potent objects, often animals or plants, that serve to define groups and identities—both in and of themselves and in contrast to those of others. For a hypothetical example, those who share the totem of the bear become united with each other as members of the bear clan. As bear-clan members, they are also differentiated from wolf-clan members—and from fox-clan and beaver-clan members. Moreover, as part of this unification and differentiation, members of a totemic group are often thought to share a fundamental nature with their totem: they are thought to possess some of the qualities of bears, wolves, foxes, or beavers. This relationship of intimacy between clan members and their totem is frequently reflected in dietary practices that prohibit clan members from killing and eating their particular totem, though they may kill and eat those of other clans.

In such totemic arrangements, each distinct group (whether bear, wolf, fox, or beaver clan) is constituted in the same sort of way. Clan members have similar relationships to one another as well as to their respective totems, and the totems themselves are similar to one another in important regards. In our example, they are all similar as furry mammals. And as various species of furry mammals, they are all similar in their differences—all are comparable variations on a common theme. In this way, the differences between the assorted totems and the clans balance out: all stand side by side; none is presumed better than any other.

However, while flaps do define groups in totemic-like ways (with those who eat flaps united and distinguished from those who refuse to eat flaps), the flap-focused groups exist in a context not of equality but of hierarchy. This is a context in which the eaters tend to be people of the Third World, and the refusers tend to be people of the First World. The meaning of totemic eating or not eating shifts under such circumstances: being unable to eat bear meat because one is a member of the bear clan is not the same as refusing to eat flaps because the meat is not good enough for one to eat. The differences between the eaters and the refusers do not balance out, and they come to rankle. Many of the flap eaters know that they are eating what others reject because they have decidedly less efficacy in the world. In fact, they fear that they are often seen by the flap refusers as being in a different and lesser league.

The rhetoric of the market might seem to dispel this fear. Thus, many meat traders (and others in New Zealand and Australia to whom we spoke) explain the primary difference between flap eaters and flap refusers not in terms of categorical difference, but as a function of relative wealth and thus of market position. They argue that in a marketplace where all sorts of goods jostle for attention and acceptance, some consumers will choose the lower-priced cuts; others, the legs, loins, and Frenched racks. But flaps are, we think, not just governed by supply and demand as these play out in relative prices and strategic choices. After all, many people in the First World can choose to reject flaps resoundingly— as not good enough for them—regardless of their financial resources and regardless of the price. Those in the Third World who cannot easily choose to reject them thereby incorporate food that others regard as intrinsically inferior, as no good at all (except for a dog).

When such a compromised commodity comes to index a whole group of people, it marks not only relative wealth and market position, but also social and economic class. That people in the Third World eat such a product resonates with their other life circumstances and prospects. For instance, many who eat flaps may, in complex ways, be more vulnerable to serious lifestyle diseases, and their vulnerability may be compounded by limited educational and employment opportunities.[54] The difference, thus, between flap eaters and refusers is not just a matter of degree— relative wealth and market position—reflected in choice of commodities. It is a matter of kind, of how a whole category of people is significantly constrained. In this regard flaps are not just another commodity circulating in the market: as cheap fatty meat deemed second-rate, flaps resist what Karl Marx called the "fetishization" of commodities.

Viewing the value of commodities simply as the price they can bring on the market—as the result of supply and demand—is, Marx argued, to fetishize them. It is to ascribe to them an autonomy—a life—of their own. It is to convey that an object has an inherent value to which people are subjectively drawn. The problem with this—with, for instance, becoming mesmerized with the diamond engagement rings in a jeweler's display case—is that it draws attention away from the labor that brings commodities into existence and which, Marx believed, is the real source of their value.[55] To ignore this labor value is to ignore the life circumstances of those who labor, which are often of enduring inequality. Such would be the case with diamond miners, traders, and cutters—not to mention the likes of factory workers—who, through various types of coercion (if only that most must sell their labor to survive), have their labor appropriated as "surplus value." This is to say, their labor is turned into a commodity for sale on the market for the profit of others. Yet it seems to us that flaps are commodities that resist such fetishization. As a cheap, fatty, undesirable cut of meat, the material nature of flaps gives some people pause: in so doing, flaps evoke the labor processes of killing and dismembering that went into them.

Flaps resist fetishization in another way, one revealed by analysis, not of what it takes to produce a commodity, but of what it takes to consume it.[56] Some analysts emphasize the efforts of advertisers to convince consumers that particular commodities are especially attractive. Others emphasize the efforts of consumers to seek out those special commodities that can best reflect and enhance their positions in the world.[57] Regardless of emphasis, all of these consumption-oriented analysts agree that once commodities become desirable, they get caught up in the construction and enhancement of identities. (For example, your car, whether a Chevy, BMW, or Prius, comes to reflect who you are, or may want to be.) Moreover, once some commodities become fetishized as better than others, they may pass on their value, their potency, to those who possess them—who themselves become fetishized as more compelling. The reverse is also true as fetishized people pass on their potency to the things they own. The lives and possessions of these compelling people become the focus of emulation through consumption: others want to be like them and therefore buy what they think such people possess. Yet, it seems to us that flaps are commodities that resist this fetishization, too. As a cheap, fatty, stigmatized cut of meat, the social distribution of flaps gives some people pause: in so doing, flaps evoke the numerous and persisting inequalities between eaters and refusers.

In effect, because lamb and mutton flaps catch people up in strongly felt likes, dislikes, or ambivalences, many of them begin to recognize—and to scrutinize—the often fraught regional relationships that move flaps from one place and group to another.[58] Flaps encourage people to think critically about the broader historical relationships that make them, for instance, into Third World eaters or First World eschewers. Thus, by following the flow of this fatty flesh from First World pastures and pens in New Zealand and Australia to the Third World's plates and pots in various Pacific Island countries, we can learn much not only about how certain societies and economies are linked but also about how people understand and experience who they are—and who they might become.

But before we can continue this flap-focused exploration of global processes as they play out in this region, we must first explain how flaps came to be: how, as one meat trader put it, they became "liberated" from sheep carcasses for sale on the market.

TWO **Making Flaps**

It may be true that meat never goes uneaten when the price becomes right. And it may also be true that lamb and mutton flaps, as food and as fatty meat, have more intrinsic value than many manufactured commodities. Yet, as we have suggested, their circulation on an international market is not a simple matter of straightforward supply and demand. After all, such circulation involves (among other things) the appropriation of surplus value and the emulation through consumption of what may be seen as the good life of modern meat eating. Thus lamb and mutton flaps (like all things that are made, sold, and bought) must be understood with respect to the social, economic, and cultural relationships—both historical and contemporary—that have made them available and, at least to some people, desirable. Moreover, because their traffic into the Pacific Islands has become so controversial, many caught up in the trade—even those who desire flaps—view them critically as embodiments of these relationships: totems standing for unequal groups characterized by differences not only in degree, but also in kind.

However, before flaps could begin to act as such totems on an international market, they had to exist as a particular sort of edible thing—as a food with a stigmatized identity, as a fatty by-product good enough for some but not others. After all, no one grows a sheep for its flaps. In this chapter, we tell their story, focusing on the history of the meat business in New Zealand and Australia and its effect on the growing, killing, and cutting of sheep.

SOME HISTORY

As we began our conversations about flaps with people in the meat industry, most told us that we could not understand the contemporary situation without knowing something about the history of the business. And just about everyone thought that New Zealand's Ross Finlayson would be an especially good person to talk with about this history because he was, perhaps, the greatest sheep-meat transactor of all time. Once called "the Kissinger of the meat industry for his frequent negotiation trips," he remains famous for having put together spectacular deals: between 1982 and 1985 he sold eleven million carcasses, or one hundred and thirty thousand tons, of mutton and lamb to the Soviet Union, filling some fifty ships.[1] Although he is now retired, he invited us to meet with him at his very comfortable home overlooking the sound in the Auckland suburb of Milford. There he told us about his deals in the context of the history of New Zealand's meat trade.

Perhaps ironically, Finlayson's great triumph was made possible because by the 1970s the New Zealand sheep-meat industry, and the New Zealand economy more generally, was experiencing increasing trouble. The picture Finlayson presented (confirmed by virtually everyone we talked with) was of extreme and ultimately unfeasible regulation. The government, working together with the Meat Board (a powerful statutory body representing farmers' interests), had implemented a thicket of measures to foster and protect New Zealand's meat exports, the country's most important source of export revenue.[2] By shielding meat processors (or slaughterhouses) from competition and assisting farmers with subsidies and price supports,[3] the Meat Board sought to keep the level of meat exports high. Under these circumstances, farmers maximized income by churning out animals, regardless of quality. One farmer described this policy to us as promoting "as many arseholes per acre" as possible. However, not only were the expenses of subsidies and price supports escalating, but the market for New Zealand's sheep meat was changing.[4]

In particular, the United Kingdom, which had traditionally purchased most of New Zealand's kill, had become unwilling to absorb New Zealand's production, particularly as sheep numbers rose and meat quality fell. This put pressure on the New Zealand processors to find new international markets. But the big meat-processing companies, Finlayson told us, had little international marketing expertise. They sought the help of independent traders, such as those at his company, Amalgamated Marketing, to sell their surplus. These traders, who were smart, crafty, and willing to take risks, were happy to help. But their efforts were not enough. New Zealand was producing too many sheep—and too many of the wrong kind: small and poorly developed animals not favored by increasingly affluent and discriminating consumers, whether in the United Kingdom or in America and Japan, New Zealand's secondary markets.[5]

Moreover, not only were British tastes changing, but so were British import policies. As a prerequisite to its entry into the European Economic Community in 1973 (now the European Union), the United Kingdom had to reach new arrangements with former trading partners on behalf of itself and the other member countries. New Zealand would be allowed to export 226,000 tons of sheep meat into the United Kingdom and elsewhere in Europe. This was considered a generous quota and was the result of effective negotiation, though it covered far less than what New Zealand was producing.

Thus, the surfeit of difficult-to-sell animals continued to grow. In desperation, the Meat Board took control of—in essence, bought—all of

New Zealand's sheep meat for two years. This control began in 1982 and lasted through 1984, at which time the number of New Zealand's live sheep reached its all-time peak of seventy million. The Meat Board first attempted to drive the price of sheep meat up by stockpiling carcasses so as to limit supplies and hence raise demand. This strategy proved ineffective. The Board then sought to unload the rapidly accumulating supply by working through existing exporters, including those in Finlayson's company, who not only acquired their meat at bargain rates but were paid a commission on sales. This strategy proved extremely costly to the board. We were told that at this time it was losing a million dollars a day and remained desperate to unload carcasses.

Contemporary traders, Finlayson said, shake their heads in recalling this period of paternalistic mismanagement. How, they wonder, could anyone have believed that stockpiling carcasses would significantly drive the price up, given alternative sources of both sheep meat and other proteins? And why had no one considered seriously the costs and logistics of storing the carcasses? The country was bound to run out of freezer space. When it did, there were suggestions that ships should be filled with carcasses and sent down to the Antarctic. Nonetheless, Finlayson, as a good trader, was able to work this circumstance to his advantage. He was able to get all the carcasses he needed, at a very reasonable price, for his huge Soviet deals.

Finlayson explained that Amalgamated Marketing owned a fertilizer business and had been buying potash from Russia, so when the Soviets became interested in buying meat, Amalgamated was a name they knew. Finlayson had always liked the Russians. He found them easy to talk to—about sports, about families—and their sociability played to another of his strong suits, at least when he was younger and weighed more: his capacity to out-drink the Russian negotiators. The whole meat-trading business, both then and now, revolves around relationships among people who know one another. The fifty shipments of sheep carcasses that he sent to Russia involved forty-five visits to Moscow over the course of fifteen years between 1970 and 1985.

Finlayson recounted the story of the last of these shipments—the last of his Russian deals:

I got on with the Russians because I never let them down. And eventually we began to trust each other enough to let each side sort out problems by itself. The last shipment was for 6.5 thousand tons—one entire ship. There it was in the Bosporus, heading toward the Black Sea, when I got a telex saying that they weren't prepared to accept it. They said that the meat had been frozen too long—longer than the agreed number of days. In fact, it wasn't any different from the rest of the meat, and no one had objected before. So I had to cope. I got on a plane and on arrival said to the boss of the importing agency I was dealing with that they simply had to take this mutton; it couldn't go anywhere else, and the only other thing to do with it was to dump it in the Mediterranean, and wouldn't that be a scandal. The boss, who always used the phrase "my dear," said, "My dear, I don't care what you do with it. I have a friend who was just shot for irregularities in a contract he negotiated and I don't want to be shot." I couldn't argue with that but asked what should be done. "Well, my dear, I think you should go home." But I told him that the ship would be in port in two days. "Go home and we'll see what we can do." So I went home and got a phone call that a telex was waiting for me at the office. The situation, it seems, had been reviewed, and they would accept the shipment for no payment, and it would be fed to prisoners. Since I was getting the meat from the Meat Board, which was in an oversupply situation, it didn't matter much. I simply told the Meat Board that there was nothing to be done. But between you and me, there was no way that the meat was given to prisoners. It was just added to the supply and became a big payoff to the Russians.

The last shipment notwithstanding, Finlayson had been very successful. Yet, although he prided himself on his trading skills, he knew that no one (himself included) could make such spectacular deals now. Whereas he obtained the meat he needed easily and cheaply from the Meat Board, today's independent traders have to acquire meat directly from processing plants—which now have their own teams of traders— and under conditions of usually limited supply. The turnabout was long in coming, but eventually the government and Meat Board were unable to sustain the system of subsidies and price supports. Indeed, with the election in 1984 of a Labour government, wholesale deregulation ensued practically overnight through the rapid implementation of a series of neoliberal reforms.

Specifically, the government ceased providing farm subsidies and abandoned regulations restricting the licensing of new processing plants.[6] These changes catapulted farmers into crisis. Without subsidies, they were forced to cut back on all expenses. Many, for example, stopped fertilizing their pastures until quality visibly decreased.[7] They also had to change farming practices and learn to grow the kinds of sheep the market desired rather than the maximum number of sheep they could. Those who could not adapt went bankrupt and sold out. Processing plants also experienced a shake-out. Some failed, some revamped, some new ones opened. All—both producers and processors—had to change practices to become more efficient in a competitive export market focused on an increasingly affluent and discriminating clientele.

In Australia, too, neoliberal reforms, though enacted later and more gradually, had decisive effects on sheep-meat exports. Australia's heavily subsidized, production-driven sheep industry was shifting to a nonsubsidized, market-driven one,[8] although in this case the flock had been supported since the 1970s in order to protect the wool rather than the meat industry. But by 1991 the "wool reserve price scheme" collapsed, and many farmers switched from growing sheep to growing wheat, leading to a reduction in sheep numbers by more than 30 percent. The regulatory changes also led to a partial shift in the kinds of sheep that were being raised. Formerly, sheep had been of merino stock, adapted not only to produce high-quality wool, but also to survive the harsh, dry climate of much of Australia. These were bigger, leggier, rangier, and fatter sheep— less good for eating—than those in New Zealand. (One Australian trader joked that New Zealand sheep are lazy because they are never far away from food in their lush green environment.) With the collapse of wool prices, not only did sheep numbers decrease, but breeds also shifted somewhat as the industry moved more into meat production, especially in better-watered coastal areas. This has come to mean that, currently, Australia and New Zealand are producing comparable animals under comparable conditions for much the same market. Still, New Zealand does remain the world's largest exporter of sheep meat, exporting 90 percent of its lamb kill, for instance, versus Australia's 40 percent—a difference partially reflecting the fact that Australia's domestic market is much larger.

Finally, and most important for our flap-focused story, there was a convergence between the New Zealand and Australian meat industries. This convergence was the product of the themes and forces that Finlayson and others saw as central to the meat history we were asking about, and it involved the cutting of carcasses. Formerly, processors had converted live animals into carcasses and left it to butcher shops to cut those carcasses into components. Increasingly, processors began doing both.

In New Zealand, meat processors first began cutting carcasses into components to profit from the change in trade agreements with the United Kingdom. Limited, as we have said, to sending 226,000 tons to the European Union (EU), New Zealand producers found that it was more profitable to fill that quota not with whole carcasses, but with the particular cuts like lamb legs and loins that would command a market premium. In Australia, meat processors never expected to profit from trade agreements, since Australia's EU quota was only 7,500 tons. Rather, they wanted to profit, by means of more efficient production, from the growing demand by Australian supermarkets (which were increasingly taking over meat sales from butcher shops) for the more desirable cuts. Eventually, New Zealand supermarkets followed Australian ones, and Australian exporters followed New Zealand ones. With meat processors elsewhere, it was much the same. Worldwide, the trade in carcasses has almost entirely shifted to one in cuts that can be distributed to the places of highest demand—with, for example, legs and lamb flaps going to—and coming to mark—different locations.[9]

WORKING MEAT

The international trade in meat begins on the farm. We interviewed a handful of New Zealand sheep farmers for this project, and we have read widely on the subject of New Zealand and Australian agriculture.[10] We learned about types of environment, kinds of grasses, methods of pasture maintenance, and breeds of sheep. We also learned about different sorts of sheep farmers. We spoke to those who viewed their farming as increasingly a technical, office-focused business—one that uses satellite imaging and computer programs to manage pasture conditions and project flock size and that relies on hired labor to do most of the physical work. We spoke to others who still run their farms as traditional, family operations, managing their pastures and flocks much as they always have and also doing much of the physical work themselves. There were other contrasts as well. Some farmers, for instance, were breeding and growing sheep for particular markets (and belonged to organizations like the "heavy lamb trust," which caters to the American preference for large but lean cuts). Others thought that conventional sheep would continue to serve them well. Despite such differences, all of them clearly recognized that they would have to survive in a world of market-based constraints. They paid close attention to market prices and frequently hedged their bets by raising subsidiary species, such as deer and cattle. All were concerned that when their animals had reached optimal size or had depleted their forage, they would find "kill-space" at processing plants.

We were enticed by what we were learning about and from these farmers, but we also realized that our project of following the flaps would become unmanageable should we venture too far down the farm lane. If we were to plunge too deeply into the world of sheep farmers—and those upon whom they relied for computer software, agro-chemicals, breeding stock, and the like—we might find it difficult ever to surface in the Pacific Islands. But it was not just for reasons of available research time and energy that we decided to concentrate more on what happens in the processing plant and beyond once sheep leave the farm.

Our desire to understand how flaps find themselves in the Pacific Islands also corresponded to the priorities of the traders whose business it is to export those flaps along with other cuts of meat. Although traders may know about farm practices (some, for instance, had grown up on farms), their most salient competency is their knowledge of how meat is processed and the many ways in which carcasses can be cut. All have visited processing plants, and many have had hands-on experience with carcasses, either in processing plants or in butcher shops. One trader told us of a meat-industry management-training program in which he spent a year rotating through various meat-processing positions in a plant.

So important was this experience to his success as a trader that, with his encouragement, his son had taken a three-month course cutting up carcasses on a meat-processing line before joining his father in business.

. . . . .

For most observers, including the traders, processing plants are charged environments. No matter how antiseptic and rationalized the procedures of industrialized killing, cutting, and packing have become, slaughterhouses are places of slaughter: they are places of fear, blood, excrement, and hot flesh; they are places of fast-paced, repetitive, and potentially hazardous labor involving implements designed for rapid dismembering. And they do not ordinarily welcome members of the public.

In his 1906 novel *The Jungle*, Upton Sinclair described American slaughterhouses as a workers' hell inhabited by immigrants with limited English and few alternative employment opportunities. Nonetheless, these workers did not take ill-treatment passively, and during the late nineteenth and early twentieth centuries "meat packing was the most strike-prone of all American industries."[11] The U.S. industry still relies heavily on immigrant labor, although the groups have shifted from Eastern European to Hispanic and Southeast Asian, and the frequency of industrial action has diminished as labor unions have lost power.[12] Certainly many social scientists, such as Donald Stull and Michael Broadway, think that in America the "human price" of meat remains far too high.[13]

Our readings about Australia suggest that the human price is high there as well. A report to the Australian Government in 1994 described employment turnover rates as high as 55 percent and concluded that it was difficult to attract "quality labour due to the poor image of the industry." Throughout the report were statements such as these: "the meat industry has been characterized by high levels of industrial unrest; abattoirs are unpleasant and dangerous places in which to work"; "the meat industry has one of the worst records for occupational health and safety claims . . . sprains and strains are the most commonly occurring injuries in the industry, closely followed by lacerations and cuts."[14]

Our conversations in New Zealand, whether with plant managers or slaughtermen, suggested that processing meat is certainly demanding work, much of it done by the most poorly educated. Yet a number of people we talked to, including traders, plant managers, and farmers, thought that labor unions once held too much power in the country's processing plants. They told us of the bad old days when thinly justified strikes, usually at the peak of the killing season, had threatened the viability of the industry. However, with the neoliberal reforms of the 1980s, culminating in the Employment Contracts Act of 1991, the power shifted decisively from the unions to management. As the term "contracts" implies, the act "encouraged direct negotiations between employer and worker, removing the special status of the union as a bargaining agent."[15] Nevertheless, even some of those who objected to labor's past power told us that the shift had gone too far, leading to the exploitation of workers.[16]

To explore labor's official perspective, we met with Graeme Cook, Secretary of the Meat and Related Trades of Aotearoa union.[17] Early in our interview, we asked him about a statement he had made, that "whipping the guts out of 3,200 sheep or 400 cattle a day is filthy, soul-destroying, boring and dangerous."[18] This was true, he said, adding that with the decline of union power in New Zealand, circumstances have even worsened. Agreed-upon terms and conditions have been eroded; the number of hours worked has increased; overtime rates (time and a half and double time) have been curtailed. The accident compensation system has been privatized to the detriment of the workers. Still, he said, working conditions are without a doubt better in New Zealand than in the United States, where the volume of kill and the speed of work are much greater and where workplace safety standards are less stringently enforced. As a case in point, he referred to a U.S. poultry plant fire in 1991 in North Carolina in which many workers died (in fact, 25 died and 54 were injured) because the exit doors were locked.[19] Such a blatant breaking of the rules would just not have happened in New Zealand.

Cook could recall only two fatal industrial accidents in recent years. Most New Zealand fatalities in meat works are due not to industrial accidents, but to heart attacks and work-related stress. The greatest problem comes from repetitive stress injuries. But there are other complaints.

Whereas in the past workers were allowed to see their own doctors when injured, now they have to see company doctors. And "Lo and behold, the company doctor is more interested in company profits than he is in worker welfare." Keeping injured workers on the job—"managing their illnesses"—cuts down on company costs: a plant gets money back from the government, much like a tax return, if only a few workers are reported injured. So, for example, one woman who had carpal tunnel operations on each wrist had to report at the plant the next day. Another who suffered a repetitive motion injury in one arm was assigned to work using the other one.

There has also been a shift in the structure of work. Cook explained,

> When I was a mutton slaughterman in the late 1980s, the day was 480 minutes long. The first work run was for 135 minutes; the second, for 110; the third, 135; and the fourth, 55. Between the second and the third runs there would be an unpaid lunch break of an hour. Between the first and second and the third and forth, there would be fifteen-minute, paid "smoko" breaks. And sometimes, depending on the union agreement, there would be an additional five minutes between the first, second, and third runs when workers would hose off the blood. Now the work day is 600 minutes—with five runs and a lunch break of only 30 minutes. It's become a 10-hour day of very demanding labor. And though most plants work their employees hard, some are really terrible. While many will, for example, use 80 workers to process 2,500 sheep, a few will use 60 workers to process 3,500. Although it was always the plant that would determine how many carcasses could be processed during each run, union members would have stopwatches to prevent bosses from ticking rates up. But the union has lost control of speeds, and workers have been unable to resist.

Cook told us about a labor dispute with a large, multiplant processing company that did not permit workers to go to the toilet. The union printed up posters showing a toilet branded with the company's logo through which a diagonal cross-out line had been drawn. In response, the company took the union to court for using its logo and won—with the result that the union was ordered to tear down the signs (which it did only partially!). The toilet issue has been significant in Australia as well: during

2002, the Australasian Meat Industry Employees Union filed a dispute notification charging that meat workers at several plants were docked about A\$3.65 for taking ten minutes in the toilet.[20]

All of these inequities are exacerbated by the fact that many plants are trying to get Immigration to authorize the importation of workers from countries with skilled cutters, such as Mexico, Uruguay, and Brazil. They argue that local labor is unavailable (as is the case with plants in Australia that wish to hire temporary migrant laborers).[21] But Cook thinks that there would be plenty of labor (even in New Zealand, where there is full employment) if wages and working conditions were sufficient. And some companies have no trouble getting or keeping workers because they pay higher wages than their employees could earn in other trades.

It is true that meat works in rural areas do have more difficulty attracting employees. But they moved to these areas for many of the same reasons that meat works have moved outside of Chicago in the United States: to get cheaper labor, to find workers who are not union-oriented. Cook said that one rural employer—in his view the worst, the least moral in New Zealand—had just persuaded Immigration to allow him to bring ten migrant workers from the Pacific Islands, and he has applied for another ten. This person, says Cook, thinks that being a good employer means taking your workers out for a few beers on Friday night. He has the highest labor turnover of any meat processor: he pays no superannuation, no penal rates, no weekly minimum, no shift allowances, no extra pay for working during holidays. And because the plant is in such a remote location, workers often have to commute an hour from home to work.

Shortly after our interview with Cook—and while mulling over his account of rural exploitation—we heard about quite a different and innovative plant. Though also rural, Canterbury Meat Processors (CMP) was said to be strongly committed to retaining its eight hundred employees, many of whom are Pacific Islanders already resident in New Zealand. We visited CMP near the small South Island town of Ashburton and spoke with Sharon McDonald, the Human Resource Manager, and with Andy Hill, the former Human Resource Manager (now working in the plant as coordinator of "Lamb Further Processing"). Both mentioned that it is, in fact, difficult to attract workers to the meat works, especially because the meat industry has changed over the past twenty years. The industry has become "mean"—the pace of the work has accelerated, and there is more pressure on everyone. CMP does try to extend a man's working life by having, for instance, more frequent and extensive rotations to allow workers to use different muscles. Yet processing between 10,000 and 45,000 lambs a week (depending on the season) is still hard work—especially at a speed of 8.5/minute along a killing line and at 8.5–9.5/minute in the boning room. "Let's face it, the meat industry is not for the fainthearted," Hill said. And it's also seasonal work. People are laid off for between eight and thirteen weeks every year. Although even the lowest-level employees can earn NZ$40,000–50,000 in ten months,[22] it's still difficult for them to make an adequate living (and, although the company never insists that people take double shifts, many are often interested in overtime work). Since there is only a 1.5 percent unemployment rate in New Zealand, CMP has to make an effort to seek out and retain workers.

The management, therefore, decided to work out a new recruitment strategy. First it sent a team to Blenhein, where a plant was closing, and offered the laid-off workers jobs. But these efforts were not as successful as had been hoped. A bit later Hill and several other CMP staff happened to be at a rugby game in Wellington. It occurred to them that they might attract workers from a local processing plant that was known to pay badly. Hill elaborated,

> We saw a lot of their guys playing and thought it might be good to run our ads down here, stay the weekend, and see what happened. In the ads we asked people whether they wanted to trade in their old lives for quieter ones. We ended up interviewing 300 people and hiring 40 to 50. They weren't all experienced. Most were Pacific Islanders—especially Rarotongans [because Rarotongans can enter New Zealand freely, without visas] and a few Samoans. We also hired a few Maori. And we got some Rumanians and Zimbabweans. Today about 30 percent of our work force is other than white Kiwi, and I don't see any problem if it goes a lot higher, as much as 70 percent.

Some of these workers are single men, but many came with families. Housing has proven to be a real problem, especially for those with large families, but the company made a special effort to make sure that the families have settled in, paying special attention to the wives, some of whom do not speak English. We want them to "put down roots," said Hill. The company has begun literacy and numeracy courses, not only to ensure the workers' safety in the plant (to make sure, for example, that they can read and understand all instructions), but also to help them advance in society. These classes take place after working hours, and they involve a huge commitment from employees who work long shifts: depending on how many animals need processing, the day shift runs from 5:30 A.M. (when workers start togging up) to 3:30 P.M., while the night shift runs from 3:00 P.M. to 2:30 A.M. Yet the classes, which involve another two or three hours a week for participants, are always filled. The company has also started a "qualification educational program" to provide "level 2 qualifications" (which allow workers to fill more technically demanding jobs, such as that of machine operator). Forty-five signed up for this, and forty will likely complete it. Hill said that these people "are going to be very proud; they will be able to say to their kids, 'Look what I have.' It is a credential they can use to get jobs anywhere."

In addition to offering courses, the company tries hard to find workers jobs in the off-season—mostly in the dairy industry, which has its busy period when the meat works has its down-time. It also sends a car to pick up workers in town, since the plant is located about nine miles away, and provides loans of up to NZ$2,000 for anyone who wishes to buy a car.

Hill did grant that Ashburton has undergone considerable change because of the presence of these new workers.

> When they moved to Ashburton, they experienced a fair amount of animosity. There was a fair amount of culture shock for everyone. It was hard for everyone to adjust. The Pacific Islanders had never experienced a small town and missed the bright lights; Ashburtons had always lived where everybody knew everybody else. In all fairness, we didn't prepare either the Pacific Islanders or the local people well enough. It wasn't until after we hired them that we met with the people who would have to be

concerned with them outside of work, with representatives from the schools and from the town council. It was a learning curve for everyone.

McDonald picked up the story. With the arrival of the Pacific Islanders, the white population at the local college (the equivalent to an American high school) declined from about 94 percent to about 86 percent—a shift that upset some residents. However, the town's initial reservations have given away to tolerance as, according to a local newspaper article, people have "accepted that . . . [the town is] growing, it's changing, and it's multicultural."[23] For example, people like the fact that one Maori family has recently opened a shop in town that sells hangi-cooked food (food cooked in an earth oven). "People living in Auckland may have had this opportunity [to enjoy this food], but few here did," said McDonald. "And now we also have taro and other interesting vegetables in our stores. I think it's very desirable if our workers find Ashburton attractive. I want them to love this place, to become integrated into the community, to enlighten the community." Hill agreed that the current recruiting experiment has been successful:

> We got excellent workers who have experienced lots of joy. We hired one brother, and then another one came, and we hired him, too. People like it here because they find it cheap to live, and so whole families move down. When they lived in places like Wellington, they never had time to see their kids play sports—and these kids would end up in street gangs. That doesn't happen here. And if a man is happy at home, he will be happy at work. CMP is like a car which will break down if it doesn't have oil; our people are like oil to us. We have to look after our people, and we want them to be happy.

We spoke to no workers at CMP and so cannot verify if they are happy or not. ("Lots of joy" strikes us as perhaps hyperbolic.) We do not know whether the educational initiatives will bring long-term benefits either to workers or to CMP. Nor do we know what will come of Ashburton's venture into multiculturalism. Who will be expected to learn what? Based on our previous research with middle-class white people who had to forge a community with Papua New Guineans, we suspect that many in Ashburton would feel that it was up to the Pacific Islanders and Maori to become more like them, not vice versa. Although tolerant Ashburtonians might come to enjoy taro in an occasional meal or a dinner prepared in an earth oven, would they be willing to do much more to adjust? What changes in the school curriculum, for example, might they accept?[24]

Rurally located CMP was innovative in its struggle to attract and retain workers, and many we spoke to considered it one of the better plants to work in. But all plants strive to keep productivity high and labor costs low. Indeed, for any plant to make meat at a profit, much must be extracted from the workers. Typically jobs in meat-processing plants are physically hard, seasonal, and not especially well paid. These jobs focus on effecting an inherently messy transformation from life to death. Workers in meat-processing plants are doing what many people accept as necessary yet wish to keep at a distance. Even the most avid carnivores among our colleagues, friends, and students feel unsettled when they confront what it takes to bring loins and legs to their tables. In fact, Sharon McDonald confided to us that she was happy to be in the front office where she did not have to think too much about the death of lambs.

LAMBS TO THE SLAUGHTER

We were able to make four visits to three small-to-medium-sized New Zealand meat-processing plants that both killed and boned animals; in addition, we made one visit to a large plant that only boned. Each of these visits required special arrangements facilitated by those who could confirm that we were not animal-rights activists or industrial spies.[25] All of the plants handled both sheep and cattle. One also handled pigs and deer. Given our interest in lamb and mutton flaps, we focused primarily on the processing of sheep. This was perhaps fortunate, since we found it easier to witness the killing of sheep—even of lambs— than of cattle, since sheep live up to their reputation for docility as they follow one another to the slaughter. Correspondingly, we could readily understand when several workers told us that they found pigs (with their humanlike cries) and calves (with their extreme youth) more troubling to deal with, at least at first.

For our main example of what goes on, let us describe a visit to a small/medium-sized plant on New Zealand's South Island. Blue Sky kills and processes up to 4,400 sheep (primarily lambs) per day in two shifts along a single (dis)assembly line. (Australian plants are similarly organized but may, like some New Zealand plants, operate several lines at once, especially during the peak killing season in the autumn.) It was the last plant we visited, and so our eyes and questions were well-focused, and our guide, the plant manager, was happy to spend as much time with us as we needed. In preparation for the tour, we put on white coats, hair nets, rubber boots, and clear plastic ponchos. We went through a foot bath and washed our hands. The plant manager asked if we had any sores on our hands or faces, or if we had a bad cough. Any of these would have precluded our taking the tour. We were instructed not to touch any surface, since this would violate various requirements of the European Union and the United States Department of Agriculture (USDA). (The manager later complained that both the European Union and the USDA are far more stringent in their regulation of New Zealand plants than they are of their own.) Then he took us to the beginning of the killing line.

Unlike most plants in New Zealand, this one does not kill in accordance with Islamic law so as to render the meat *halal*—suitable for Muslims. That is to say, the sheep, once rendered unconscious by electrical stunning, do not have their throats cut by a ritual practitioner.[26] Most New Zealand plants, we had already learned, slaughter in the halal fashion: lucrative Middle Eastern markets require this, and markets elsewhere rarely object. However, the farmers providing sheep to Blue Sky (a company with substantial farmer shareholding) are staunch Presbyterians and do not want their "Christian" sheep subject to Islamic procedures.

At this non-halal and state-of-the-art plant (opened in 1987), sheep are simply electrocuted. They then tumble through a chute to enter the "slaughter board and dressing chain." From then on, the carcass is handled on an assembly line. Workers, the great majority of whom are not only men, but large men (many, indeed, are Maori and resident Samoans, Tongans, and other Pacific Islanders), engage in a variety of fast-moving, strenuous operations (sometimes rotating tasks with their immediate neighbors). The death of animals becomes a series of matter-of-fact operations to make the animals edible and profitable.

The first step is to attach each dead sheep to an overhead rail along which it moves down the line for processing. Hung initially by both forelegs and a back leg with head upward, the animal has its throat cut open first. Then, after moving along an electrified bar—to stimulate and then relax muscles so as to reduce twitching and facilitate handling—a worker thrusts a hooked knife into the opened throat, cutting the major vein (the vena clava) and releasing a torrent of blood. As the carcass moves along the line, other workers plug its anus and remove its hoofs (using hydraulic hock cutters). The dangling head is clipped off, and the carcass is shifted so that it is held by just its front legs. Then the pelt is removed in a series of operations that involve slicing along the front legs to open it up, loosening it across the upper chest, and then, with machine-operated clamps, pulling it down to the upper torso. Using a special knife to avoid spilling the guts, the workers split the pelt open at the belly. At this point, a hydraulic ram with a smooth paddle is slipped inside the front-opened pelt to separate the skin from the carcass so that it hangs loose. Grasped from below by a machine, the pelt is pulled off the lower legs like a pair of trousers and falls into a receptacle to be sold for further processing. (In plants without these pelt-separating machines, the process is far more laborious. For instance, the skin must be separated from the carcass by a man who forces his fist repeatedly between the skin and the carcass, a particularly strenuous procedure known as "punching down.")

The next job involves lifting out the guts and the offal, snipping open the chest with large hydraulic shears, and removing the lungs. These innards are placed in trays moving along a belt next to the line: guts in one, edible offal (such as heart, liver, kidneys, sweetbreads, and sometimes tongues and brains) in another, and inedible offal (such as lungs) in a third. At the same time, meat inspectors are checking each carcass as it moves by. If they find that an animal had a serious disease, they pull it and its corresponding innards off the line. Cosmetic flaws, such as bruised portions, are dealt with at this point through excision. Finally, at the end of the line, a grader weighs and tags each carcass. In addition to recording the weight, the tag, which is applied to the carcass's Achilles tendon, indicates the "mob" number (assigned to the farmer for his particular lot of sheep) and the grade describing the carcass's quality. Occasionally, if the animal was obviously too fat, the tag also indicates its "GR"—the Greville measurement of fat—which reduces the carcass's value.

At this point, the processing on the slaughter board and dressing chain is complete. With the exception of the flaps, all of the low-value elements have been stripped from the carcass. The pelts are destined for fellmongeries, where the skins and the wool will be processed further. The blood, feet, and assorted leftovers are sent to rendering works, where they will be converted into a range of products including tallow and meal. The inedible offal (as well as any pieces that may have fallen on the floor) goes to plants that make pet food. The edible offal is shunted aside for packaging, freezing, and sale as such. Though all of these parts are by-products in the sense that no one raises a sheep in order to produce them, they do have a value that must be realized if the processing plant and those they buy from and sell to are to make a profit.

The carcass is then prepared for the next stage, where it will be cut into marketable pieces. Still hooked to the overhead rail, it must first go through an accelerated conditioning tunnel, where it receives additional electrical stimulation to further relax muscle fibers. This procedure, together with temperature control, greatly speeds up the aging process necessary for the production of tender meat. Then the carcass is conveyed into the chiller, where it is grouped with others of comparable size, to be pulled out as needed for processing. Once the flesh is chilled enough to become firm, accurate cutting can begin in the boning room.

In the boning room the major cuts—those producing the "primals"—are made with a bandsaw. A worker grabs a carcass off the rail, flops it down on a bench, and slides it against about 2.5 feet of exposed blade.

He cuts the carcass horizontally into approximate thirds. The first cut is made through the base of the spine so as to remove the still-joined back legs. The second cut is made between the shoulder and the middle section. Next the worker splits the middle section along the spine into two pieces. (Recall that the front of this section had already been cut through when the lungs were removed.) Finally, cutting each of these middle pieces lengthwise, he separates the back from the belly: the high-value loins and racks from the low-value flaps. (It is this processing that is reflected in the diagram of lamb cuts in the introduction.)

Significantly, flaps are the only parts of the carcass that do not get further processing. Like pelts and offal, they are by-products—the residuum of the carcass—to be stripped out of the way to facilitate the extraction of higher-value cuts. Therefore, flaps are shunted off to the side at this point, placed in plastic bags, and laid in sturdy, waxed cardboard cartons (measuring about 52×40×18cm and weighing approximately 20 kg). The cartons will be frozen to at least minus 18°C for shipping to clients.

The rest of the dismembered carcass continues down the conveyer belt for further splitting and for expert cutting by "boners." With remarkable speed and dexterity—knife in the cutting hand, chain-mailed glove on the meat-holding hand—they trim the racks, "bone out" the shoulders to sell as roasts, dissect the legs to sell as silverside, thick flank, topside, and rump. The cut and boned pieces are diverted to various packing stations, where they are prepared for shipping. Unlike the flaps, which are simply stuffed into bags, these cuts are likely to be individually wrapped before they are frozen or chilled, so that each piece is protected from the vicissitudes of travel and conveniently packaged for use in hotel and restaurant kitchens or in supermarket displays. It is assumed that clients interested in such cuts—as opposed to those who buy lamb and mutton flaps—expect that their meat has received such careful treatment. Not only are flaps rather unceremoniously stuffed into bags and thence into cartons when processed, they often are simply band-sawed into halves or quarters when they are sold, or they are cut into slices of about three-quarters of an inch thick.

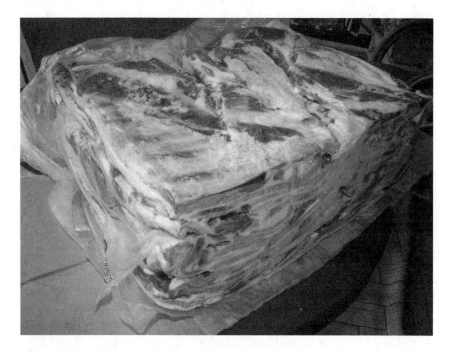

Figure 3.   Flaps, just out of the half-carton

THE AMBIGUITIES OF FLAPS

Even though no one grows—or kills—a sheep for its flaps, the cartons leaving the factory must find a destination in order to contribute their 3–5 percent of the carcass's value. But they do carry something of a stigma, particularly in the Pacific Islands where, as we have said, they function as totems that both mark and create the unequal groups—the eaters and the refusers—for whom they are either good enough or not good enough to consume. As such, their comings and goings refuse to be fetishized as simply a matter of supply and demand. Because of their particular material attributes as cheap, fatty by-products, they resist such fetishization: they remind people of the processes of killing and dismembering that produced them; they remind people of the numerous and persisting differences between eaters and refusers. That is, they compel all of those caught up in their trade to scrutinize the fraught regional relationships that move flaps from one place and group to another.

As cheap meat, flaps will (as the New Zealand trader told us) readily circulate in a market. Indeed, from the point of view of their processors, flaps must find buyers because no profit can be made until all parts of the sheep are sold. As fatty meat, from the point of view of their consumers, flaps have the capacity not only to nourish but to over-nourish—and thus contribute to serious diseases. As we have said, many health professionals think this trade in flaps has had a role in creating unhealthy Pacific Island bodies, since diets high in animal fat contribute to obesity, hypertension, heart disease, and diabetes. And they agree that, while these diseases have been on the rise worldwide, they have risen dramatically in some Pacific Island countries.[27]

But, in addition to their capacity both to nourish and to over-nourish, flaps have other ambiguous attributes. As by-products, they are never produced for their own sake. Moreover, flaps lie ambiguously between the cheap fatty meats that constitute world-traversing, highly caloric, branded and patented fast foods (like McDonald's hamburgers and Kentucky Fried Chicken pieces) and the cheap fatty meats that constitute the regionally distinct, highly caloric, ethnic foods (like Italian "lardo" and Afro-American "chitlins").[28] Unlike the first, flaps do not evoke an imagined international community of flap-eaters. After all, many Pacific Islanders know that flaps are by-products that white people refuse to eat. Nor, unlike the second, do flaps (yet) generally evoke a valued way of life. Many Pacific Islanders also know that they are a recent introduction from elsewhere.[29]

Such ambiguities are both expressed and compounded in what is, perhaps, the major wrangle concerning Pacific Island relationships: whether or not lamb and mutton flaps are *dumped* by regional First World countries on Third World countries. A 2002 newspaper article written by the Asia-Pacific correspondent to the British newspaper the *Independent*, for example, articulated themes subsequently reiterated in the international press after the death of the King of Tonga, whose obituaries frequently described him as the world's most enormous monarch, the leader of "a nation where coconut flesh and mutton flaps are dietary staples."[30]

Pacific Islanders' Fatal Diet Blamed on Kiwi Exports

Only the choicest cuts of New Zealand lamb find their way to European dinner tables. A very different type of meat—a fatty offcut called mutton flap—is exported to the South Pacific, where it contributes markedly to the region's dire health problems.

Mutton flap, known locally as "sipi", has become a staple protein in poor Pacific nations. While islanders regard it as a delicacy, governments have condemned New Zealand for "dumping" the inferior meat. The Prime Minister of Tonga, Ulukalala Lavaka Ata, dismissed it recently as "hardly edible".

Tonga is threatening to ban sipi—chunks of bone and fat cut off the end of top-quality chops. Also exported from Australia, it forms part of a diet blamed for the Pacific's alarmingly high rates of obesity, diabetes and heart disease. Fiji outlawed mutton flaps in 1999 [actually, in 2000].

New Zealand's Health Minister, Annette King, said it would be "morally imperious" to dictate what other countries ate. Meat producers said they were merely meeting demand. . . .

Sipi is just one type of low-grade meat exported to the Pacific, in a practice that Rod Jackson, professor of epidemiology at Auckland University, calls "dietary genocide." . . .

A fellow epidemiologist, Robert Scragg, was equally scathing. "Australia and New Zealand have made a big song and dance over the years about French nuclear testing," he said. "Mutton flaps have caused more deaths in the Pacific than 30 years of nuclear tests."

New Zealand is paying a price, however. Many Pacific Islanders exploit family links in Auckland to seek costly dialysis treatment. Medical bills are often left unpaid—and the government is threatening now to clamp down.[31]

As the article makes clear, accusations of "dumping" (allied with references to dietary genocide and nuclear contamination) are often efforts to disambiguate flaps so that they appear as fundamentally irredeemable, as ill-suited for human consumption. Relying on the overlap between the alimentary images evoked by the verb "to dump," the accusations are efforts to insist that the trade in flaps (and other fatty meats) be appraised and regulated, not just in commercial, but also in moral terms. Technically, as used to describe trade, dumped flaps would be those that enter the market as the result of (some sort of) subsidy and, because of this unfair advantage, skew the appropriate conditions of competition—perhaps eventually reducing consumer choice.[32] But in these accusations, dumping does not refer to an unfair advantage in the market economy, but to an unfair advantage in the moral economy. And yet, as the New Zealand Minister of Health said, to dictate what those in other countries can choose to eat might be seen as "morally imperious."

Thus, by virtue of their (persisting) ambiguities, flaps are good to think about and good to argue with. They are complex and are perceived in contradictory ways. As fatty flesh, they can nourish; as fatty flesh, they can over-nourish and produce fatty flesh. They are delicacies for the Third World, and they are hardly edible by-products (some, as we shall see, say they are waste products) from the First World. They sustain free trade and incite banning.

THREE Trading Meat

New Zealand and Australian traders who sell meat to consumers in the Pacific Islands bristle at stories like the one we just presented about the King of Tonga. They do not want the publicity, they told us. They do not want the interference, they are not greedy, and they are not looking for the kind of deals Ross Finlayson made with the Soviets. That world, they believe, was never truly viable because it was not based on market forces. Their world involves smaller margins (3 percent if everything goes well) for lots of work, lots of knowledge, and lots of risk-taking. They just want to do their jobs, and these, they say, are crucial to an important industry and to people around the world who need food they can afford. They complain that flaps and those who trade them into the Pacific Islands are unfairly singled out, since many other high-fat foods, like corned beef and butter, are being traded into the Pacific Islands. The focus on flaps also overlooks the fact that there are many protein products from all over the world traded into the Pacific Islands: Chilean tuna, Chinese luncheon meat, Australian chicken parts, and U.S. chicken wings canned in China. And even if people do get sick from eating too many flaps, the traders are not responsible for their behavior. In addition, flaps are quite different from the bottom-of-the-line sheep scraps that are made into a slurry, pressed and frozen into blocks, and sold to Ralston Purina in the United States for use in pet food. The meat world is complex and competitive, and traders know it well. They do a lot for the money they earn.

In this chapter we present the perspective of these men in more detail (the meat trade is overwhelmingly the domain of men).[1] Although ideologically we are not the free marketers they are, we found them engaging, enterprising, outgoing, and curious. In some ways, they are the commercial corollary of anthropologists. Just as anthropologists have their cognitive maps depicting where and why certain peoples favor staples like taro or tapioca, traders have their maps showing where and why certain peoples favor, or might come to favor, particular cuts of meat. Once processors began to cut carcasses into components for which markets were needed, they had to configure the world in a more ethnographically detailed way. One trader, for instance, told us that in his effort to find new markets, he first went to South Auckland to see what Pacific Islanders living there were buying in the shops. Based on this visit—a sort of field trip—he concluded correctly that those still living at home in the Islands would probably like flaps and other cheap, fatty cuts. Moreover, like anthropologists, traders take pride in their ability to orient themselves in different sociocultural situations and to engage with a range of differently located people. And, like anthropologists, they enjoy telling vivid stories about the adventures they have had and the people they have met.[2]

IN THE OFFICE

Not everyone in the meat trade bothers with the Pacific Island market (or with other marginal or emerging ones). Yet everyone in the contemporary meat industry is preoccupied with moving meat, and there is much meat available for sale to these markets. The clogged freezers and stagnant cash flow that gave Finlayson his Soviet deal are the opposite of today's "best practices." The largest meat processors are preoccupied with selling large volumes as efficiently as possible, and while the volumes processed by the medium and smaller firms are not as great (a fact that some of their salespeople may find slightly liberating), the smaller firms certainly have to be efficient as well.

Many processing firms move meat through their own traders, who either sell directly to clients or to independent traders who have their own clients.[3] Some firms—usually the bigger ones—employ one of their traders to sell into the Pacific Islands. The trader (usually a junior member of the firm) tends to engage only with more lucrative and reliable clients, such as those in the high-volume supermarket trade in Fiji or the high-value hotel trade in Tahiti, who can be expected to pay relatively promptly. Conversely, processing firms are reluctant to bother with markets that are in any way risky, requiring extensive local knowledge or close monitoring. Therefore, as one independent trader explained, "they leave it to us to sell difficult products to difficult markets."

Independent traders often like such a challenge. They think of themselves as really good at selling, at finding a market, at knowing a range of products. To be sure, a background in the meat industry is useful. A background in business more generally may also be useful. And many have worked in export firms. But what really counts is having a trading spirit and being a quick learner—being able to make the most of opportunities in a business with "a steep learning curve."[4] In fact, many independent traders distinguish themselves sharply from those they see as more narrowly focused specialists working for huge firms, who spend their days "behind banks of computers buying and selling 65cl beef [cheap hamburger]."[5]

We started our work with these independent traders by consulting a pamphlet produced by Meat and Wool New Zealand, *The Business of New Zealand Meat*,[6] which lists the 136 processors and exporters licensed in the country. We were most interested in those businesses whose major markets were reported as comprising, for example, "Papua New Guinea, Fiji, Tahiti, Tonga, Samoa, and all other Pacific Island destinations" and whose major products include "chilled/frozen lamb, mutton, beef, venison, and variety meats [offal] plus meat and bone meal, fish meal, and tallow."[7] We soon learned, however, that even these relatively specialized companies trade many more products far more broadly when opportunities arise.

Our strategy was to telephone the directors or marketing managers of these companies, explaining as quickly and persuasively as we could that we were interested in changing foodways in the Pacific, that we had long-term research experience in the region, and that we had worked, as well, with a major multinational corporation whose directors found us discreet and fair. (This was the British-based firm, Booker Tate, which had managed Ramu Sugar Limited.) If they asked for more specifics, we acknowledged that we were interested primarily in the trade in lamb and mutton flaps. We stressed, though, that we had no axe to grind concerning this trade and, indeed, had known many Papua New Guineans who benefited nutritionally from eating them occasionally. (We also mentioned that our book on flaps would not be coming out any time soon, a fact that many seemed to find comforting.)

Given the controversy surrounding the trade in flaps—especially Fiji's ban and the possibility of future bans elsewhere—it was no wonder that several of these traders were initially dubious. One wanted to know whether our interest in flaps was "political"—likely to create unwanted publicity. Another said that he did not want conversations that might in any way unsettle his relations with his clients—indicating that a difficult market had been made more difficult by the controversy over flaps. In addition, they wished to protect commercially sensitive material from competitors. Yet by assuring them of our discretion—that we would be careful in our conversations with other traders, in public statements, and in our writings—and by incrementally building contacts and, hence, credibility, we were able to meet with representatives of most of the independent companies either currently or formerly trading into the Pacific Islands.

One appointment generally led to several others as traders recommended us to their New Zealand and Australian colleagues, both those who work independently and those who work for a processor. Often they could give us their colleagues' telephone numbers from memory or by quickly checking the automatic dial listings on their own phones. Traders do form something of a loose community, even though it is a community of rivals. Most either know or know about the rest, whether in New Zealand or in Australia. They may have once worked in the same office as another trader or know someone else who had. Traders do cooperate across firms on occasion—as in negotiating shipping rates or in warning about untrustworthy overseas clients.[8] They recognize that in their relatively small world people move around, and things come round. Today's competitor may be tomorrow's ally and vice versa. Therefore, one generally should avoid "cutting another's lunch" (undercutting another's almost completed deal). But however friendly they are, traders in one company do not expect to be friends with those in another.

These traders seemed to find our questions—framed most broadly as "What do you have to know to be good at your business?" and more specifically, "What do you need to know to sell lamb and mutton flaps to Pacific Islanders?"—sufficiently engaging to spend at least several hours with us in their offices. (This, despite the fact that they are, as we will see, very busy—if not traveling, then catching up, keeping in touch, pursuing prospects.) In some cases these office interviews led to repeat visits and after-hours socializing. Several told us that they had never been asked by anyone to describe their skills in the meat trade. Indeed, some joked that they found our interest a refreshing contrast to the attitudes of their children, who were often reluctant to discuss with their friends what their fathers did for a living.

One independent trader explained that the "essence" of what he and the other independent traders do is to add value—both for those from whom they buy and those to whom they sell:

I take on the difficult tasks for packers [processors] in dealing with markets that they may be unfamiliar with. I also help importers, by sorting out prices. I know that the world market is soft and falling. I know that a product might be cheaper tomorrow. I know when a product is likely to be sold out, when it has gone to Timbuktu [just disappeared]. And I know from importers when there is an oversupply in their markets. In many markets importers take positions and make mistakes. They buy two, three months in advance and want to lock up the market. And I pass this information on to packers. Sometimes, though, I will tell packers that you are selling too cheap—that you can get more money for your product. They know I am giving them information that will help them. And it won't undercut the customers who already bought from me. [These customers would be undercut only if their competitors got the same product at a cheaper price.] I sit in the middle. It took me three years to realize that I could help both sides, and once I realized this, my company took off. Now I leave most of the trading to the others in my firm [there are five] and spend my time at the computer, checking exchange rates, trying to make money on the currencies we buy and sell in.

Like the other offices we visited, his was usually buzzing. And like the others, it had an "open" office plan in which traders, each tending to focus on a set of clients within a particular region (such as China, Mexico, Korea, or the Pacific Islands), sat near to one another so that they could readily share information about which products were available and at what prices.[9]

This is how a New Zealand trader described a normal day:

I am usually in the building before my boss. I'll turn on my computer and, as e-mails are getting downloaded, will check for faxes. Fewer and fewer come in since e-mails are much better because they provide you with an instant record and you can reply instantly. And then I'll just set about the day. I'll often get a hundred e-mails. . . . Then I work from there: I talk to meat packers; I make inquiries; I begin speculating. A trader never has nothing to do. I will e-mail people and learn that a supplier will have a certain number of flaps, and I'll begin costing them off. I'll e-mail Samoa and make an offer as the day progresses. Different prices come in. I look at them. I know if there is an excess of volume on the market. I know that I won't be able to move them at a particular cost. From my sources in Fiji I know the prices things are moving for. They will tell me that this stuff is selling at this price. I check on the exchange rates. And then I will begin to cost backwards—to figure out what the price would have to be [and in what currency] for me to sell it there and make my margin. And sometimes just keeping in touch pays off.

This trader, in calling around, was able to get a good deal on twelve forty-foot containers of size 11 chickens (smallish chickens, weighing 1.1 kg), which he sold to Fiji. It happened this way: "An Australian company, Inghams [primarily a chicken producer], was lucky enough to get the KFC [Kentucky Fried Chicken] chicken contract for all of Australasia. Though it was great for Inghams, it was also something of a mixed blessing because there is always 'fall-out,' which KFC doesn't want. I knew a guy at KFC who was an ex-meat trader, and he told me about it all and talked to people at Inghams and was able to help make the deal."

Another New Zealand trader—whose goal is to develop trade in all sorts of foods throughout the Third World—had also been busy pricing chickens. He has been sourcing chicken leg quarters from the United States for sale in the Pacific, as they have become cheaper than "turkey tails" (another very fatty meat popular among Pacific Islanders).[10]

> Chicken had been 30 to 60 cents a pound, delivered, but the price had dropped to 27½ cents a pound. And the freight component is somewhere between 11 and 14 cents. This is cheap chicken [which is to say it only costs about .13/lb to buy]. I think that people in the U.S. have lost the key to the chicken-production factories, or that the machine is locked, and they just keep pumping them out. The feed must be pretty sophisticated, and producers have gotten the idea that they should grow anything they want. But I lost money when the price suddenly went up. Everything I buy has been "forward bought" [pre-sold]. And I had promised to deliver a certain amount of chicken at a certain date. But I got burned when the U.S. government decided to buy a lot of chicken for school lunch programs and to feed prisoners. The market had been just sitting around waiting for these announcements, and I got caught. It happens.

In fact, he got caught again, although in a somewhat different way, concerning fish from Chile in the aftermath of the 2004 tsunami.

> Chilean fish suppliers suddenly got a huge order for canned fish as tsunami aid for Indonesians who couldn't fish for themselves because their fishing areas had been torn up and polluted with bodies. A billion cartons

were sent to the relief effort. And then everyone, including me, expected that there would be a good fishing season in Chile from February to July, but this just didn't happen. So I couldn't fulfill the orders for my clients in Samoa. I could have fulfilled the order of one, but not both—and since these guys are big rivals, they wouldn't share a container. So I sent to neither. If I had offended either one, I would have lost him. So I'm hedging my bets. I might lose them both—and if I do, it will affect my sales of flaps and other meat. I'm just on the phone all the time, constantly massaging people so as to maintain my market. And then there's the problem of getting paid.

The big processing companies stay out of such micro-level massaging, often by staying out of certain markets entirely. They do not want delayed payment, and they especially do not want to act as bankers for clients who cannot pay until they themselves have sold the product. They also do not want to help their clients with customs obligations or to get involved in sorting out difficulties about the overseas whereabouts and fortunes of a lone refrigerated container.

We learned of one such container when we visited the office of an independent firm for a follow-up interview. Holding twenty-three tons of the firm's frozen meat, it was sitting on a ship beached on the Mexican coast. In between transactions, traders searched the Web for information, including news from a site operated by a local maritime enthusiast who was posting pictures of the ship as events unfolded. (The cause of the accident remained unclear because the captain had disappeared.) The traders quickly learned that the ship could not be pulled off the sandbar. Battered by the waves, it was listing heavily and leaking oil. But were its generators still running, sending power to the cooling units of the refrigerated containers? Several days passed before they knew that this was the case. Finally, just as the ship appeared to be breaking up, a heavy crane was brought to the scene. But even if their container were rescued, what would be the fate of its perishable contents under the Mexican sun? Would there be electricity on the beach? And who would take charge?

Eventually the news came that the container was safely off the ship and properly plugged in. Two members of the firm, already traveling on business in Mexico, together with an insurance agent, were there to open it. Everyone was greatly relieved that the meat was still frozen and that the refrigeration log showed that there had been no significant interruption of power. They certainly did not want insurance wrangles and disappointed clients.

Although being in the middle does demand considerable micro-massaging, traders can sometimes be not only conciliatory but also forceful. We caught one Australian trader in a particularly forceful mode as he was continually interrupted with pressing phone calls during our interview. These involved three issues. The first concerned a lawsuit he had brought against a former employee who had stolen his "intellectual property" by copying client lists and other materials from the office computers in order to start his own trading firm. The second concerned an East Indian who sells rubber gloves in Papua New Guinea. Somehow he had decided to try his hand at selling meat and had ordered a container of Australian lamb necks from a New Zealand firm. He was unable to sell them himself and so, the trader explained,

I am willing to buy it, but this guy must continue to pay the power costs and the interest on the amount he borrowed to buy the stuff. The last thing I need now is a container filled with necks. I think this guy is just trying to fuck me around. And I'm the one trying to be responsible to the marketplace! If this guy keeps the necks, he will have to sell them for next to nothing, and then the price of square-cut shoulders [another cheap cut, though one more expensive than necks] will go down, and everything will collapse.

The third pressing issue involved several calls to and from a meat processor concerning freight incentives. These are incentives to the meat processor to load shipping containers so that they are as full as possible when they leave his plant. The trader explained this between phone calls:

The more that is loaded, the less per kilogram of shipping costs—since you are paying for the container, for the fork lifts, for every action on the docks. On the other hand, the less that is loaded, the more per kilogram you will pay. There's a leeway on each side, but once it is five hundred kilograms in either direction, incentives cut in. This guy had tried to sell me flaps at too high a price. I told him I wouldn't pay and made him a counteroffer. One of the calls I just took was him saying OK but that he didn't want to be docked for under-filling a container. Bullshit. He's just trying to make trouble. He's just a cheap bastard. He calls up and says, "Please, please, please, take my stuff" and then turns around and wants you to pay immediately.

Meat trading, hence, especially by independent traders, is intense. Remaining on top of this game requires vigor, persistence, concentration, strategy, nerve, charm, and toughness. These traits, one trader told us, are exactly those of a good salesman. A successful trader has an energy level higher than most, gets on with people, and has cunning but also integrity. Being in the middle—adding value for everyone—means understanding both product and market. It means "keeping the talk going and being willing to bluff, if necessary." But it also means that you have to come through, or else you lose it all.

Making a living by getting flaps and the like to those who want to buy them at a competitive price is very demanding. Hence, most traders think they do not have the time—much less the responsibility—to worry whether such meats are too fatty to be good for Pacific Islanders who choose to eat them. Indeed, they regard the charges of dumping not only as misguided and unfortunate but as adding insult to injury, given the exigencies of the Pacific Island trade.

OUT OF THE OFFICE AND THROUGH THE PACIFIC ISLANDS

In our discussion with the great meat transactor Ross Finlayson about the history of the trade, he mentioned that his deals in the Pacific Islands (mostly in Samoa, Tonga, and Fiji), though initially auspicious, often went sour. Just when traders were scrambling to open up new niches for carcass components in the Pacific Islands, the markets there were becoming much less dependable.

At first, throughout the Pacific Islands, traders had been able to rely on a set of stable clients: large, long-established, European-owned, and, to a lesser extent, Asian-owned, firms that operated with an "indent" system. They knew their own local, substantially expatriate, demand and simply placed routine orders with the same Australian and New Zealand exporters. If these orders were filled at a reasonably good price, everyone was happy. In effect, as an Australian trader told us, "Everybody could remain in their comfort zones and still make money." However, the big expatriate-owned firms with their largely expatriate clientele—all with strong ties to the mother countries—are mostly a thing of the past. Only a few substantial firms remain, some owned by Asians, some by Europeans who may be married to Pacific Islanders, and some by indigenous businessmen (who, in Fiji, tend to be Indo-Fijians). But there are also many smaller, indigenously owned firms, and these constitute the primary market for the independent traders, since the larger firms, if they pay promptly, may be able to buy directly from processing plants. And for many traders, including Finlayson, dealing with these smaller firms has become difficult indeed.

As Finlayson told us, "These people have absolutely no concept of paying." Some of his firm's worst debts came from Samoa. After a somewhat unknown (but promising) client was allowed to run up far too much debt, Finlayson was sent to collect. Although he was at that time a very large man himself, the delinquent Samoan storekeeper behind the counter was even larger. Finlayson explained that there was a problem with the account: namely, that his firm was owed two hundred thousand dollars. The storekeeper responded by placing a huge knife on the counter and saying, "Well, I can't pay you because I have this fishing boat to run." Finlayson replied, "Well, what are we going to do about that fact?" And the storekeeper said, "We aren't going to do anything about it."

We were told a similar story about Samoa from a trader no longer selling to the Pacific Islands. Promising to tell it to us as it really was, he wryly recounted some of his business dealings there.

They had no understanding of business, no understanding of money. We would sit around a table, and there would be a hundred dollars on it; I thought that this would be part of the payment for the product I had brought. And they said, "No, no, let's share it." I was sending about eight to ten containers a month of brisket, chicken leg quarters, corned beef, povi [brined brisket], flaps, and turkey tails—most of which ended up at the church. These people have a feast in church every week. And people from the church weren't paying for the stuff when they went to the store to get it. They were putting down a deposit of something worthless—an old electric jug, a broken-down car. Products would disappear, and no money would come back. Then when you went to the churches to complain, the preachers would say it was all done for God. . . .

One Samoan shopkeeper used to cry to me all of the time that his business was terrible and that he wasn't getting any money. Well, I sat down and said, look, we have sent you this and this, this brisket, and you are pumping up the price by 40 percent; where is all of your money going? Well, I learned that he had a relative who was a politician and that he himself was chief of the village and so had to share with everyone in the village. So, if he made a thousand dollars, only a third of it would actually go to him. I know that he was under huge pressures to share. People now have huge families since there's better medical care. And, another thing, they have to keep giving to these churches. I was at one church, and there was a listing of what people had given. One family gave a thousand dollars. Another family, two hundred dollars. A third, nothing. People lost face if they didn't give and would be ringing up their kids living abroad to send money to help them. One thing is sure: none of that money went to me. I once took my lawyer with me to collect, but that went nowhere. I wouldn't consider doing business there again unless I or one of my people were there all of the time.

We heard comparable stories about other markets within the Pacific Islands. One trader referred to Tonga as an economic Chernobyl, a place he has "whited out" on his map of viable markets because he could never collect what he was owed. And those who pulled out of Papua New Guinea cited problems of default as a major reason (along with those of law and order). Fiji, with its internationally oriented Indo-Fijian businessmen, was something of an exception. But even there, payment was far from automatic. One trader found that his Indo-Fijian clients were more likely to pay up if he went round with a large indigenous

Fijian male of military background and bearing. Another hired an asser-
tive Indo-Fijian woman to scold and shame her male co-ethnics into
settling their debts.

.   .   .   .   .

What, then, does it take to be successful in such a generally difficult
market? In talking to a number of New Zealand and Australian traders
still active in the Pacific Islands, we gathered the following.

Traders must really know how to sell to this specialized market. The
trade has become very demanding—hands-on and competitive, lean
and mean. Traders must leave their offices and dive into multiple worlds.
With clients from the better-established stores, they attempt to nurture
long-term ties through regular visits and holiday gifts. Traders may also
nurture relationships with their long-term clients by filling special—
often improvised and decidedly heterogeneous—and not necessarily profitable orders. Thus, along with meat and other provisions, one
trader filled a client's request for a used Holden transmission.[11] Another
trader complied with a client's request that his next container include a
carton of his favorite, hard-to-find pickled herring. Traders also provide
other services to cultivate their networks, both present and future. They
may, for instance, meet a client's son or daughter at the Sydney or Auckland airport to buy the child lunch and make sure the connecting flight
to boarding school is met.

It is much more difficult to cultivate long-term relationships with owners of the smaller, indigenously owned stores—as the stories we have related about Samoa indicate. The smaller stores frequently go under. They
tend to be undercapitalized and disorganized, and thus especially vulnerable to substantial overhead costs stemming from, for instance, the
demands of kin and church, and also from robbery and various other
forms of default. In dealing with these stores, traders must temper their
eagerness to chase up orders with a realization that it may be hard to
chase down debtors. Certainly, with the smaller stores, traders expect to
extend credit beyond the conventional thirty-day period (after delivery)
to forty-five and often to sixty days. In effect, traders recognize that they

must act as bankers to these clients—waiting until the clients sell their stock before paying for it. When visiting these clients, traders look closely for signs of whether the business is going downhill: Is the store busy with commerce? Is the owner in attendance? Are clerks responsive? Is the store well stocked? Are there containers with additional stock in the yard? If not—and if other suppliers say that they have not been paid in a long time—it may be time to cut back or to retreat entirely. Of course, it would be preferable if they did stay in business. In fact, it is sensible for a trader to do what he can to make sure, as one told us, that "everyone makes a few bucks along the way."

Protecting one's commercial interests in such a firsthand manner requires skill not only in appraising particular operations but also in being sufficiently rough, ready, and resourceful—having enough vitality and savvy—to negotiate the features of the Pacific Island scene more generally. All of those we know—especially those who traded into Papua New Guinea (where law-and-order problems may be especially serious)— prided themselves on their stamina, both emotional and physical. They could cope, as one had to, when mugged in the parking lot of a major supermarket. They could deal, as another was forced to, when his twenty-foot shipping container of flaps was hijacked on its way into the Highlands by villagers who hacked it open with axes. They could manage, as yet another was compelled to, when his visit to a store was cut short by an approaching riot.

One trader told us that he really enjoys the adventure of selling meat into Papua New Guinea. He sometimes feels that he is "going back in time" to the very beginning of outside influence, of commerce. He is excited to be in a country where flaps have been, until very recently, a wonderful novelty for many. To work in what he saw as a frontier-like trade, he developed a special strategy. In addition to cultivating clients and coping with circumstances, he has created his own contingency force. On his visits throughout the country, he establishes and maintains collegial relationships with police commanders and their senior officers. He buys them drinks and dinner, and presents them with souvenir police badges acquired from the Auckland police force; delighted, the Papua New Guinea police complete the connection with the Auckland force by giving him badges in return. Above and beyond whatever enjoyment the trader derives from the company of Papua New Guinea cops, he knows that they will try to look after his physical safety. Moreover, if a defaulting client seeks to protect his resources by fleeing to his home village, the police will travel there, "knock a few heads and scare up some payment." (This trader told us that he even likes telling stories about how tough it is to do business in Papua New Guinea because it scares off prospective competitors.)

Another trader said that he enjoys the challenge of mastering the Papua New Guinea market. At least in one case, this involved him in a field project of sorts. He decided to supplement his visits to shops with a trip to a Papua New Guinea rubbish dump. In this way he could learn not only about what was for sale, but also about what was actually purchased. At the dump, he noted with interest the preponderance of small packages of gum and cigarettes and small cans of meat and fish. From this, he deduced that Papua New Guineans are not interested in economies of scale. Not only do they lack the ready money, but they also would rather not be cleaned out of any leftovers by improvident and importuning relatives. Thus there would be little point in trying to persuade them, for instance, that a leg of lamb might actually convey more value for the money than flaps.

This trader also used this insight into the Papua New Guinea market as well as his special skills as a trader to augment his trade in flaps and stay one step ahead of the competition. (He describes himself as a "dead-meat man," coming from a long line of butchers, who can "visualize a carcass" better than anyone so as to create new kinds of cuts for sale.) He knew that while whole pigs' heads were readily available for export, there was only limited demand for them in Papua New Guinea, despite the well-known liking for pork there. The limited demand seemed to stem from two factors. The first was obvious: a domestic pig industry was protected by a 70 percent tariff on imported pork. The second seemed related to his observation at the dump: a pig's head was too large and too expensive to be purchased casually. The trader's solution was to innovate. He arranged with his meat processors to slice the very fatty jowls from the heads as a separate cut, producing pieces that were then of a suitable size to be purchased readily. They were also inexpensive because they could be imported duty-free.[12] Designated as offal, they have been exempt from the usual tariff on pork.[13]

However, traders into the Pacific Islands know that none of these coping mechanisms or innovations would matter unless they could offer competitive prices and services—and they must be quite competitive since Pacific Island firms tend to serve a customer base of very price-conscious clients.

In fact, most traders into the Pacific Islands agree that trade there is not only difficult and (sometimes) dangerous but generally too narrowly focused on "commodities" to be fully satisfactory. Traders recognize, of course, that everything for sale in the meat business is, strictly speaking, a commodity. But some products—those they term *commodities*—are heavily price-driven. That is, when products like flaps are standardized, usually available, and cheap, clients generally decide to buy from one trader or another primarily according to narrow differences in price.[14] Clients rarely develop much loyalty to any particular trader, so that traders must compete hard for clients on the basis of cost, making profit margins slim. The result is that if traders are to make a profit in the Pacific Islands, they have to work hard to control costs, anticipate risks, and move high volumes. Some can get good at this and make a lot of money; but even they can get tired of selling just "commodities."

Most would like to sell higher-value products—and not just because these tend to be more profitable. They would like to be able to work with their clients to develop their market—to encourage greater sophistication in their customers and expand their sales from flaps to necks, chops, and legs (if not racks!). In so doing, traders and clients would develop ongoing relationships—mutual commitments that transcend, at least somewhat, the precise price of a product at a particular moment. In addition, such relationships would depend on, and validate, the full range of a trader's knowledge about the global traffic in meat (and other products). Such relationships would enable a trader to add value by providing not only products at very good prices, but also sound advice about what and when to buy—including what new products to try. Finally, at least during introspective moments, *some* of the traders saw themselves as engaged in global trade for global benefit.[15] In fact, they wanted their Third World dealings to provide a positive impetus for the unfolding of an expanding, market-focused prosperity.[16]

Unfortunately, both for those trying only to make a buck and for those also trying to make a difference, the Pacific Islands are generally not cooperating.[17] Markets there are stagnant—not "developing." As such, their long-term economic prospects do not appear good. There is little industry, and in places like Tonga (according to the traders), most of the money spent on imports like flaps comes from remittances by overseas relatives. Sales of flaps are likely to remain flat, and markets are unlikely to diversify as traders would like them to. Traders, thus, have moved their business away from the Pacific Islands not only because they have become tired of struggling with defaulters, but also because they have become tired of selling basic products to people who will not be able to afford anything much better very soon. It is perhaps no wonder, then, that those who remain committed to the Pacific Islands may occasionally think they have made a mistake by staying on. One, claiming to have had lamb and mutton flaps on the first post–Cold War ship into Vladivostok, wondered whether he should have pursued this and other markets, which are more likely to expand and diversify.

THINKING CRITICALLY ABOUT FLAPS

The kind of world Ross Finlayson inhabited, one in which he could negotiate spectacular deals for sheep carcasses with the support of the Meat Board and a system of subsidies, has given way. Replacing it is a world that—if allowed to work properly—is envisioned as a map of niches, created and filled by knowledgeable specialists who can articulate cuts of meat with local desires and economic circumstances. In this contemporary world, cuts of meat as well as those who trade them are all subject to similar market-based standards. Whether going as loins to France or as flaps to the Pacific Islands, cuts jostle with each other in the marketplace. And whether selling loins to France or flaps to the Pacific Islands, traders jostle with each other for market share. The jostling of cuts reflects global supply and demand; the jostling of traders reflects savvy and resourcefulness in meeting that supply and demand.

To sharpen this general picture—both to focus it more sharply on the Pacific trade and to address a nagging question in our own minds—we (rather cautiously) asked a number of traders a comparative question. Was selling flaps to the Pacific Islands regarded as an inherently less desirable—less classy—business than selling more expensive cuts elsewhere? Some traders—including those who no longer concentrate on the Pacific Island trade—rather reluctantly confirmed this. Island traders were likely to be really good at their work, and they certainly had great stories to tell. But they now were really working at "the bottom of the market." Moreover, selling commodities like flaps into Papua New Guinea does not require as much sophistication as is needed, for instance, to sell the best-quality beef to Japan. Yet there was general agreement that these distinctions were relatively minor, readily offset by degree of success. One trader drew an analogy: You might have an up-market clientele and product in selling BMW's, but you could do pretty well in selling used cars. Maybe even better, and that counts for a lot.[18]

Thus, for those who do sell flaps to the Pacific Islands and prosper in the business, the primary problem, as they see it, is not that their business lacks class. It is that flaps as a commodity are problematic in other ways. Unfortunately (and unfairly), the trade has become politicized. Rather than jostling with other cuts of meat in the impersonal process of worldwide commerce, flaps have become subject to unfavorable attention—as products that some eat because they are cheap and others refuse to eat because they seem unfit for human consumption. The trade in flaps, in this way, becomes more fraught and complex than the mere working of market forces would imply. In this way trade is hindered, and traders are stigmatized.

Flaps are not only trouble, but troubling. For many analysts, observers, and consumers—although not for many traders—flaps have come to represent structural inequalities between First World producers like New Zealand and Australia and Third World customers like Pacific Islanders—inequalities that are evoked by the charges of "dumping." To label flaps as "dumped" brings both the product and those who purvey it under special scrutiny. To the extent that this scrutiny interrupts business as usual, it invites an examination of the processes of the structural difference that delimit the choices available to some and not to others; an examination of how cheap, fatty meat ends up only on certain plates and in certain bodies.

FOUR

Papua New Guinea's Flaps

When we asked traders to explain how lamb and mutton flaps ended up on Papua New Guinean plates and in Papua New Guinean bodies, many began with a general story linking the earliest contact between Europeans and Pacific Islanders with the trade in meat. According to this story, animal protein was always scarce for Pacific Islanders and hence a luxury item. Consequently, imported meat of even the cheapest kind was immediately deemed desirable, as the initial explorers, whalers, traders, and missionaries (some say Captain Cook himself) discovered when they first traded in brined brisket of beef. (Brisket is a cheap, fatty cut from the breast of a cow, about 15 percent of the animal.) The Pacific Islands were, in this rendition, the global entrepreneur's dream: a market just waiting to be tapped and one both deep and easily filled with low-quality meat products.

So successful was this trade that, in Tonga, over the many years since the first European contact, brined brisket has come to be regarded as traditional ceremonial fare. In more recently contacted Papua New Guinea, brisket has also featured in the (non-expatriate) trade. Just as Papua New Guinea was emerging as a promising market, we were told, brisket became available at a most competitive price. During the late 1970s and early 1980s, the primary markets for Australian brisket had been the United States and Canada, where it was ground into hamburger. However, both countries abruptly stopped importing brisket after discovering nodules (probably caused by midges carrying roundworm). This left Australian meat processors with a great volume of low-value beef clogging their freezers, and they looked immediately to Australia's de facto colony to the immediate north—Papua New Guinea.[1] Especially appealing were the densely populated Highland regions that were increasingly affluent (through coffee growing) and accessible (through a vastly improved road system). In the Highlands, pork was the principal protein. Highly valued, it was only rarely consumed, primarily on ceremonial occasions like weddings and funerals.

Moreover, according to the traders, Highlanders not only liked meat, they especially liked fatty meat, given the high-energy requirements of living in a relatively cold climate. It was clearly another market waiting to happen, though not as profitable as the previous one. Indeed, once nodules were no longer declared a health hazard, the brisket trade immediately shifted back to North America. Significantly, we were told, the sudden withdrawal of brisket left Papua New Guinea with "a big, gaping desire." Fortunately, another cheap meat was increasingly available in the country to fill this desire: the lamb and mutton flaps that Australia and New Zealand were now exporting in large quantities. This was what the global market was all about. As one trader put it forthrightly, "One person's trash was bound to be another's treasure."

Although Australia had the initial foothold in Papua New Guinea, New Zealand was quick to follow. Gray Mathias, a trader from New Zealand, told us about his ventures selling flaps (mostly) into the Highlands, starting in the 1970s. This populous, recently accessible, increasingly prosperous, and protein-short region was a big, new, and eager market.

> Flaps were a dirt-cheap commodity. I could get them at one time for 10–12 cents/kg. The market for flaps was underpinned by the Highlands. Especially when . . . [the big, expatriate-owned Highlands stores] began to put in freezers. Before the road was completely opened [the Highlands Highway, linking the port cities of Lae and Madang to the Highlands], hundreds of tons of the stuff were flown to the Highlands from Madang. . . . Once the road opened, I could then sell thousands of tons in the course of a year on ongoing contracts. The demand and the value followed coffee production. During the early days, this little Highland guy, all painted up, would come down from the hills with his coffee. And in half an hour you'd see him in a brand new Datsun 1200 "ute" [a pick-up truck], loaded with lamb flaps, driving home. When Collins and Leahy [one of the big expatriate firms] got their cold stores in [the Eastern Highlands town of] Goroka, they could stock, I estimate, ten thousand tons in it. . . . It was an amazing business. Sometimes I'd have four hundred tons of flaps on one ship alone. I got people to pack the stuff in white cartons, which got a premium. And then when I started using cartons with Rastafarian colors [and the four seasons depicted on them], which Papua New Guineans liked, I could get more for them. They'd use the cartons as wall paper.

The trade in flaps and other foods of modernity subsequently became much less promising.[2] In fact, in Papua New Guinea, as elsewhere in the Pacific Islands, the trade has become just plain difficult. Certainly traders trying to do business in contemporary Papua New Guinea find little to remind them of the initial entrepreneurial glory days—little of the rush from making a commercial first contact. Rather, the history of the trade has come to mirror the history of the country's development: a history of persistent, if generally unsatisfied, aspirations, of citizens finding it increasingly difficult even to make ends meet, much less live expansive lives like that of the man with his new Datsun 1200 ute. Yet, the trade in what some think of as trash and others as treasure remains substantial. During 2005, 17,214 (metric) tons of lamb and mutton flaps were exported from New Zealand and Australia to some five million Papua New Guineans (for an annual per capita consumption of about 3.4 kg).[3]

A HISTORY OF DEVELOPMENT FROM THE INSIDE

The excitement—the opening up of economic possibility—was especially intense in the Highlands. In contrast to the rest of the more accessible, if more thinly settled, parts of the country, the Highlands had come under effective colonial control only after World War II. Indeed, the Karavarans of the East New Britain Province, among whom Fred worked, and the Chambri of the East Sepik Province, among whom Deborah worked, had long been "pacified" (Karavarans since the turn of the twentieth century and Chambri since the late 1920s). Correspondingly, both were accustomed to the material objects that white people possessed and traded. Nonetheless, not just in the Highlands but throughout the country, the decade before and after national independence (in 1975) brought considerable enthusiasm about "development."

There is no doubt that our Karavaran and Chambri friends, like many Papua New Guineans at the time, were excited by the new commodities becoming available to them. Access to these things appeared to promise freedom from a colonial circumstance in which they were often depreciated both individually and collectively by white people. They would have what white people had and thus be their equals.[4] During Fred's (1968 and 1972) research, his Karavaran friends made clear that their desire to acquire "cargo"—manufactured commodities—was rooted in their long-term efforts to compel white people to recognize mutual human-ness. In particular, they referred to the "dog movement," a series of meetings held during the 1930s in which they discussed with perplexity and anger why the colonists persisted in treating them with contempt—driving them away, telling them to get out, as if they were unwelcome dogs. The contempt, they concluded, was driven by their lack of the commodities that white people so obviously valued. If only they could learn how to place an overseas order, then too their ship (literally) would come in. In fact, they did place an order through an expatriate importer for a ton of rice, ninety-five pounds of twist tobacco, twenty cases of corned beef, half a ton of sugar, and fifteen cartons of biscuits. Though they got what they paid for, they had hoped for far more—enough to narrow significantly the gap between themselves and those who looked down on them. However,

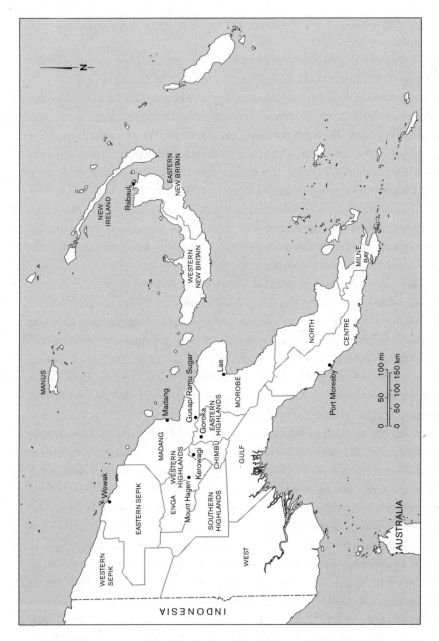

Figure 4. Map of relevant places in Papua New Guinea

they remained optimistic: development, while proving elusive, might still arrive.

This is not to say that the Karavarans or other Papua New Guineans wished for development in order to become white people. Indeed, they often thought that white people were borderline sociopaths—amoral and antisocial in their self-centered atomism.[5] Development would not mean abandoning cultural traditions and social groups. Instead, it would be an augmentation, in many respects, of what they already were, through the incorporation into their social and ceremonial lives of rice, tobacco, corned beef, sugar, biscuits, and eventually brisket and lamb and mutton flaps—even Datsun 1200 utes.

This promise of development became an impetus, not only for cash cropping (like the coffee that made Gray Mathias's business possible), but also for wage labor, much of it in the growing Papua New Guinean towns. Those receiving the best jobs were those who had the best formal, Western-style education. And so many Papua New Guineans began to fantasize that at least one child, generally a son, would become educated enough to get a job away from his village and send money home. However, although many children received schooling through the sixth grade, few passed the nationally administered standardized test with a score high enough to secure a place in the seventh grade. And fewer still overcame later hurdles.

We got a firsthand sense of the hopes and fears resting on test outcomes one evening (a bit later, during 1987). We were in a Chambri village when the test results were announced. The atypical silence throughout the village was only occasionally interrupted by localized shrieks of joy from clusters of kin, all huddled around a radio, learning that one of their children might yet acquire sufficient education to qualify for a well-paid job. Of the forty Chambri children who had been evaluated, only four made the grade. The rest, whose formal educations would likely stop, became known—and knew themselves—as "standard six drop-outs." They were disappointments. The money already spent on their school fees had been a waste because they probably would never be able to contribute much to bigger and better bride prices, bigger and better ceremonies, more and different cargo that villagers hoped for.[6] They would never be able to contribute much to the augmentation that development promised.[7]

There is no doubt that these expectations and such unequally distributed educational opportunities contributed to significant changes. Leaving the village, at least for a time, became important. Towns were, after all, both the sources and the centers of development. Many Papua New Guineans—and not just youth with prospects for further education and good jobs—felt that to spend their whole lives in villages would be to miss out. And in fact, the urban population increased in the country from 4.8 percent in 1966, to 13.1 percent in 1980, and to approximately 15.2 percent in 1990.[8] In addition, with improved roads, many people could feasibly travel to town, stay with kin, and have a good look around. Some became permanent residents who made only occasional trips back to their home villages. Others engaged in circular migration, coming and going when it was convenient. All either had mastered or were mastering a lingua franca, principally Tok Pisin, and so were able to communicate with strangers.

We wanted to learn about what life in town was like, and so, during 1987, we moved into Chambri Camp, a settlement of Chambri who had left their three home villages for the coastal town of Wewak, the capital of the East Sepik Province. By the early 1970s Chambri had been arriving there in ever-increasing numbers, and by the time we lived there the camp was well established. Some Chambri moved in with relatives. Others built houses or additions to existing structures from whatever was available—bush materials, scavenged pieces of sheet metal, and even cardboard (perhaps from lamb and mutton flap cartons!). Chambri in the camp came to describe it as the fourth Chambri village.[9] Indeed, as many lived there as in any one of the three home villages. And like Papua New Guinean migrants more generally, many of those living in the camp eventually considered town to be their primary home.

To be sure, the comings and goings of urban life could be exciting. Chambri clearly enjoyed wandering around Wewak, often in the company of Chambri friends—visiting the crowded shops, markets, bus stops, sports fields, and churches. But town life was also sometimes dangerous, as there was a high incidence of crime.[10] Moreover, since most people had little money, town life was frequently hard. Only 17 percent of adults living in Chambri Camp during 1987 had regular salaries. Most of the other men and women in the camp were artisans—carvers or basket weavers—and relied for their survival on income earned from sales. Yet during the three months of 1987 in which we collected data, many of these artisans made no sales at all. They eked out a living somehow, but they had much less food than they would have had in their home villages, where fish is always plentiful. They subsisted at least partly on smoked fish occasionally sent from kin at Chambri, green mangoes gathered from trees belonging to others, and small marsupials killed in the bush. When they had money (sometimes remittances from family members farther afield in Papua New Guinea), they generally bought the cheapest foods they could, including canned fish (increasingly from factories in Papua New Guinea), canned corned beef (also likely produced domestically), and pressed pork loaf (mostly imported). Also popular were rice and instant noodles (mostly imported), as well as local vegetables such as pumpkin tops and other greens, sweet potatoes, taro, and sago. Finally, since there were freezers in the towns, they would sometimes, as special luxuries, buy chicken parts (such as necks or even "cocktails") produced by the country's own poultry industry or (very fatty) sausages produced by local supermarkets. These foods, with the addition of lamb and mutton flaps, were the urban staples elsewhere in Papua New Guinea as well.

Partially offsetting the difficulties of town life was a sense of freedom—not only the experience of novelty but also of release from certain coercive aspects of village life. Though none of these Chambri migrants wanted to cease being Chambri, many—especially the young people—did find town liberating. One young man (quite well educated although not formally employed) said that in town "you are free to walk about; you are the master of yourself." By contrast, in the village you had to be very wary of the "ancestral custom of killing people by poisoning [ensorcelling] them" and thus take care not to offend the "big men." Chambri leaders, he elaborated, used their power to prevent the younger men and women from holding all-night dance parties to modern music because they thought that such occasions encouraged young people to choose their

own sexual and marriage partners rather than acceding to marriages arranged by their elders.

A similar view, reflecting a woman's perspective on Chambri as a
place to leave and avoid, was presented by a woman of twenty-nine. She
had been living in Wewak for seven years, supported largely by remittances from a brother working in the Bougainville copper mine (which
closed in 1988). When we asked her why she did not return to Chambri,
she at first said she was foolish for not doing so since Chambri was a
much better place than Wewak—everything in Wewak must be bought,
and one must have money simply to survive. Why then, we persisted,
did she not return? Lowering her voice, she revealed that she and many
other young women did not go home because they would be expected to
marry old men whom they did not like and would be subject to sorcery
if they refused.[11]

The life course of one of Deborah's oldest Chambri friends, Joseph
Kambukwat, illustrates vividly many of the promises and disappointments of development, much of the push and pull between village and
town. Born (we estimate) in the early 1950s, Joseph was educated at
Chambri by Catholic missionaries through grade four. Singled out for
further education by a visiting teacher from Australia, he attended a
Catholic school near Wewak. There he finished grade eight in 1968 with
a reasonable command of English. His education was interrupted by a
return to Chambri following the death of his father and the remarriage
of his mother. In 1972 he left Chambri again to attend a trade school, and
upon graduation he worked first with the National Works Department
and later with the police force. After receiving police training in Port
Moresby (the country's largest town and administrative center), Joseph
joined a Mobile Squadron located in Rabaul (another principal town).
But then he became ill. Convinced that his bad health was the result of
sorcery perpetrated by Chambri who were jealous of his good job, he
left the police force and returned to the village. In 1974, with the arrival
of Deborah at Chambri, he became her research assistant and language
teacher. In 1975 he married Elizabeth—Sapet—and the couple soon had
two children. Then Sapet fell ill, and when medicine obtained from a
medical orderly failed to cure her, Joseph again concluded that sorcery

was the real cause. Eventually, through divination, he learned the identity of the sorcerer, a man who apparently had wanted to marry Sapet himself and felt that Chambri marriage customs gave him a stronger claim on her than Joseph had.[12] Joseph tried to appease his rival with the gift of two pigs along with money and betel nut that he distributed to appropriate recipients—and Sapet did recover. Yet the couple remained uneasy; they concluded in 1981 that they would be safe only if they left Chambri. Wewak was too close to Chambri for comfort, so they moved to the somewhat more distant town of Madang. As a commercial and tourist center, Madang already hosted a sizable community of Chambri, who were engaged in producing and selling artifacts and in wage labor.

Indeed, Joseph soon was hired by the New Zealand manager of Madang Timbers, who was impressed with his command of English and a letter of recommendation from Deborah. Joseph's job was to make sure that orders were filled correctly with the right kind and dimension of lumber. Joseph liked the job—the pay was fine, the responsibility was gratifying—and he and Sapet lived happily and healthily in the company of other Chambri. Eventually he acquired his own long-term lease on a block of land from the government, to which he paid regular rent. But all of this "modernist" living ended in 1995 when Sapet died shortly after giving birth to their fourth child. In addition, Madang Timbers was sold, first to Filipinos, who cut his pay, and then to Chinese, who cut it again, demoted him, and were rude, never even saying good morning or good afternoon. They treated him, he said, like a slave. And so in 2001 he left that job and has been supporting himself ever since as an artifact carver.

Deborah had not seen Joseph since her second visit to Chambri in 1979, although they had corresponded a bit, and she knew about his move to Madang and the job with Madang Timbers. When we arrived in Madang in 2006 on this project, he was easy to find, along with other Chambri, in the section of the town market devoted to artifacts.

It was a grand reunion and an occasion for much reminiscing, even as he brought us up to date about the unhappy events that had occurred in the past few years. Over the course of many subsequent conversations,

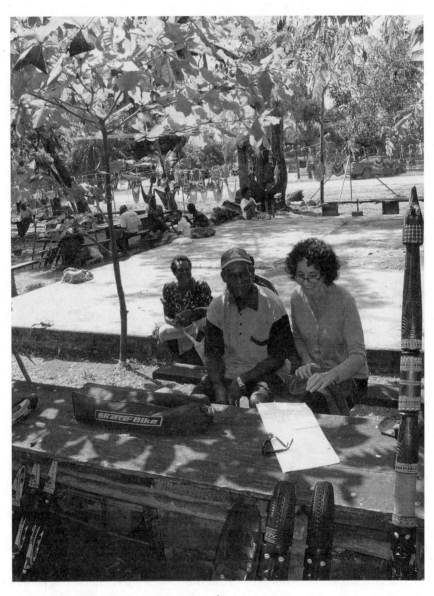

Figure 5. Joseph and Deborah at Madang's artifact market

we learned much about his recent life. Times have been hard, for him and for many people throughout the country. Money is short, the kina has fallen in value, and the prices of everything in town are way up. After Sapet died Joseph could not afford to buy baby formula; the infant, Michael, would have died too, but a kindly chemist provided formula at a huge discount. And tourism is way down, largely because of Papua New Guinea's reputation as a dangerous place. Often Joseph, who is the major breadwinner in the household, sells nothing at the market; sometimes he cannot afford the 50 toea (US$.15) bus fare and must make the long trip home on foot in the scorching tropical sun. He cannot afford the fees to send his two older children to high school, and he owes money for the younger one's tuition. Worst of all, he and his children sometimes must go without food. Although he likes chatting with his mostly Chambri neighbors in his community of Sisiak, he often is distracted by hunger, and he cannot speak of it, lest he be seen as making a request of others, who most likely are as short of food as he is. He recently had to tell Michael that he is a big boy now—too old to cry when he is hungry.

While the promises of development have faded for Joseph, he does remain committed to town life. He told us that his last visit to Chambri was more than ten years ago. His brother decided recently to return (in order to maintain control over family land), but Joseph has no thoughts of doing so. His wife is buried in Madang, and he still is angry at the way she was treated at Chambri. At Sisiak he can live with other Chambri without feeling coerced or threatened by them, and he also enjoys engaging with a wide range of other people at the market. Besides, even if the excitement of town life has worn off for him somewhat, his children cannot imagine being back in a place where nothing is happening. Indeed, since only the eldest speaks any Chambri (as most conversations among Chambri youth are conducted in Tok Pisin), it would be hard for them to live there. And education and health care are much better in town.

Joseph's experiences—like those of the other Chambri migrants we spoke with in Madang and Wewak—are of course culturally and regionally inflected. Undoubtedly those Chambri who responded to the push from traditional village life and the pull into modernist settings by moving to Highland towns such as Goroka and Mount Hagen had somewhat different experiences. However, the economic decline—the shortness of money, the fall of the kina, the rising cost of everything—has affected ordinary people throughout the entire country. One of Fred's Karavaran friends put it more strongly than most when he said (in 1991), "I will never believe in development again," but many Papua New Guineans would ruefully agree that things have not worked out as they had hoped. Getting by is harder and harder. Certainly the amazing, expansive, and exuberant era of new markets and exciting possibilities appears to be over.[13]

Yet cheap, fatty meat still has its place. As we will see in the next chapter, the vast majority of those interviewed by our Papua New Guinea research assistants reported that the reason they do eat lamb and mutton flaps is because money is short and flaps are cheap—and, for most, quite enjoyable. Not surprisingly, when Joseph bought a special meal for his family with his first pay from us, he chose the food Michael likes best: lamb and mutton flaps.

CHEAP EATS FOR HARD TIMES

We learned a great deal about the role of lamb and mutton flaps in Papua New Guinea life from the interviews with Joseph and others. However, to supplement this information, we used our connections with Chambri in Madang to find out more about the food preferences as well as actual diets of at least some of the urban poor. In particular, we focused on the two hundred Chambri (and their twenty-one in-marrying husbands or wives, coming from various parts of the country) who lived in twenty-eight houses at the Sisiak settlement during 2006. Thirty of these people had some regular income, but most of them earned only minimal amounts (nine, for example, were paid about K50/fortnight [US$16.60] working as laborers for Madang's RD tuna cannery, and two were paid a modest stipend for acting as Community Magistrates). Since we had limited time available (again, the dilemma of a multisited research strategy), we devised measures to achieve rough understandings. One measure involved Joseph's asking seventy-nine of his adult Chambri friends and neighbors (two to four adults from each household) what food they liked best and what they would buy if they had K20 (about US$6.30) to spend. We selected this amount primarily because it would seem something of a windfall, authorizing an extravagant purchase. The answers given to Joseph were the following: 30 friends would buy frozen chicken pieces, 21 would buy fresh fish, and 20 would buy lamb and mutton flaps; other answers were canned corned beef (5); eggs (1); both lamb and mutton flaps and fresh fish (1); and both canned corned beef and canned fish (1). His respondents gave a variety of reasons for their choices. One, for example, said that he liked eating lamb and mutton flaps because they are greasy and taste good when mixed with garden foods (like greens and taro) purchased at the market. Another said that he liked eating fresh fish because it is what he was brought up on at Chambri, was not too greasy, and was delicious with sago. Another preferred canned corned beef because it is ready to eat, an entire meal in itself.

We also asked five Chambri to collect information from six households (their own and, in one case, a closely related one) about what members actually ate each day. Household size varied from four to eight members—a total of thirty-four people in all. Three of these households had members who held jobs (two locally with minimal pay: one as a laborer at the RD cannery and one as a teacher at an elementary school, respectively; one as an employee at a gold mine some distance away that paid better). Our assistants collected data for two weeks, and, to avoid contaminating the survey, they were not paid until their work was concluded. We also asked Joseph, who at the time was being paid by us, to record the foods eaten by the ten people living in his house (himself, his four children, two in-marrying spouses, and three grandchildren). According to these data, a strong (and predictable) correlation exists between the kind of food eaten and the amount of money available. Unfortunately, we do not have data about how much of each kind of food was actually consumed.

The poorest household, of two adults and two children, was also the smallest. The husband worked as an artifact carver, and the wife as a basket weaver. Sales were infrequent. This family ate twice a day. Typically, in the morning they would share a pot of rice creamed with coconut milk and in the afternoon, bananas, noodles (a cheaper variety than Maggi), greens acquired at the market, and tea. Occasionally, perhaps if a sale had been made, they would add a small can of fish, fried flour balls, bread, and once, lamb and mutton flaps. The least poor household in our sample (the one headed by the gold miner, who was away during our survey) consisted of two married couples, one unemployed adolescent, two schoolchildren, and one four-year-old. People in this household also ate twice a day, but often snacked as they went about their routines. Here is a typical day of eating for the adult male artifact carver who lived in this household: in the morning he ate rice, fried onions and noodles; in the afternoon, an ice block (a popsicle) and buns bought in town; and in the evening, rice, noodles, greens, and canned fish—and sometimes, rice, noodles, greens, and lamb and mutton flaps.

Finally, there is Joseph, who, on the first day after he received money from us, began to enjoy his new affluence. In the morning he drank a Coke; in the afternoon he had bread and tea; and in the evening he ate rice, greens, noodles, lamb and mutton flaps (Michael's choice), and tea. On another occasion, in the morning he ate rice, noodles, and canned fish; and, in the evening rice, fried onions, noodles, smoked fish, and canned fish. And on yet another, in the morning he had an egg sandwich and a can of orange soda purchased in town; in the afternoon, a coconut (while waiting for a sale at the market); and in the evening, a stew made of rice and saw-mince (the fragments of meat, fat, and bone leftover when a butcher cuts meat with a bandsaw). Again, we emphasize that we do not know how much people were actually eating. But we do know from Joseph and others that they and their neighbors were often hungry. And we could see that urban Chambri of all ages were very lean. This picture was consistent with other information that we were gathering in Madang.

To learn more about what Papua New Guineans were eating, we visited the James Barnes factory, which has been producing canned corned beef in Madang since 1986. Trevor Hattersley, the expatriate financial manager, was quite forthcoming with us. The company, he said, is in real trouble. Canned corned beef is a dying industry in Papua New Guinea because times are so hard.[14] Cheap canned fish is the most popular protein, followed by lamb flaps. Canned meat is only a weak third. It is just too expensive for most Papua New Guineans because it costs so much to make. Most of Barnes's meat is imported, and droughts in Australia have driven up the price of beef, while the value of the kina has dropped. Barnes simply has to pay too much for what it imports—and this is so even though there are no tariffs on beef destined for further processing.[15]

In contrast, a can of tuna from the local RD factory is about half the price of a can of corned beef. There is some false economy here: the 400 grams RD promises you is actually somewhere between 200 and 220 grams; the rest is water and oil. When Barnes fills its cans, it does so with 420 grams of solid beef. But this does not matter to the consumers as much as price does. And in other ways as well it is hard to compete against RD.[16] The (Filipino-managed) factory was built just out of town, so it can pay its workers rural wages. Until recently, many workers were earning as little as K44/fortnight (US$14.67)—and out of that they had K9 (US$3) deducted for meals (some rice and a bit of fish), and they had to pay a transport allowance as well. They would come home with 30 kina (US$10). RD no longer charges for meals or for transport costs, but the wages are still extremely low. Moreover, the company often sacks people after three months and then hires them back to avoid providing vacation leave and retirement pay.

Barnes is experimenting with other, more cheaply produced protein products: chickpeas in brine; chickpeas in curry sauce; mexibeans; and a new idea—chicken in curry coconut cream (from locally produced chickens and coconuts). There are still a significant number of Papua New Guineans who do not have electricity and want some source of cheap, convenient protein. And the market for corned beef is not completely dead. Sales go up when there is money around—as, for instance, when it's coffee season in the Highlands. Barnes's product is about 16–18 percent fat, but that is what people here like. When the factory first opened, it made a corned beef product with about 6 percent fat, similar to one sold in Australia, that was finely minced and pressed tightly into cans. Most Australians refrigerate it, then take it out of the can and slice it. But Papua New Guineans like this chunky, fatty product that they can put on top of carbohydrates and vegetables. Still, the Barnes company is barely surviving. And now extra competition exists in the form of cheap and even fattier lamb and mutton flaps—again, 17,214 tons were imported in 2005, and annual per capita consumption is 3.4 kg.

A WORLD (SOMEWHAT) DIVIDED

What we learned from all of these Madang-focused measures and conversations is that the diets of Joseph and many other rail-thin Papua New Guineans weathering hard times are certainly nothing like the diet of the 290-pound Tongan woman we read about who eats 2 kg of lamb flaps every day (more than two hundred times the rate of Papua New Guinea flap consumption) along with other high-calorie foods. Her circumstances appear to be reflected in the health statistics from Tonga, where, it will be recalled, more than 60 percent of those aged fifteen and older are obese, 29 percent of the population dies of cardiovascular diseases, and about 15 percent (and rising) have diabetes.

The statistics from Papua New Guinea are less dire, but they are also less comprehensive and less conclusive—they are derived from studies of rather limited populations within particular areas of the country, and many were conducted some fifteen to twenty years ago.[17] Dr. Peter Siba, director of Papua New Guinea's Institute of Medical Research, told us that little work is being done in the country concerning nutrition "because today's priorities are malaria, HIV/AIDS, pneumonia, tuberculosis, women's health, and health delivery systems." Although the country is experiencing an increase in so-called lifestyle diseases, especially among civil servants who do not eat well or exercise much, "no one is doing the research which would produce the concrete data necessary to pressure the government to spend more of its resources on nutrition." Indeed, the information that is available is provocative in its ambiguity. One scattering of studies and observations does seem to reveal a circumstance of serious over-nutrition.

One often-cited survey by the International Diabetes Institute was conducted in 1991 at Koki, a relatively affluent suburb of Port Moresby inhabited for several generations by people originally from the coastal village of Wanigela (several hundred kilometers to the east). Among those from Wanigela living at Koki, 27.5 percent of the men and 33 percent of the women had diabetes. In the home village the incidence of diabetes was also high—17.9 percent among men and 10 percent among women—although significantly less so. Among villagers of another ethnic group living midway along the coast between Wanigela and Port Moresby, the diabetes rate was 1.1 percent among men and 2.8 percent among women. The Koki diabetes rate is thus vastly higher than that of any other group in Papua New Guinea, urban or rural, and the figures perhaps suggest that genetic factors as well as long-term urban residence are implicated in these extremely high numbers.[18] Still, studies show that obesity and the incidence of cardiovascular disease for men and women older than eighteen are highest overall in the National Capital District (which includes Port Moresby), and the rate has been rising.[19] Correspondingly, the proportion of patients admitted to Port Moresby General Hospital with cardiovascular disease has increased from 1 percent in 1960 to 5 percent in 1974 and to 11 percent in 1997.[20] More generally, obesity has been found to be most frequent in urban coastal areas—though still relatively rare in rural areas and in the Highlands.[21] Observers note that the dietary changes leading to chronic lifestyle diseases—dietary changes focused on consumption of fatty meats—have been most common in villages with easy access to urban centers.[22]

We also asked a physician now in private practice in Madang about his experiences with diseases of over-nutrition—diseases caused by eating too much of the "wrong kind" of food. When he first started practicing in Papua New Guinea in 1985, he said, years might pass without his seeing a patient with diabetes, and during his first five years in Madang (beginning in 1996), he hardly saw any. But during the past five years, diagnoses of diabetes have become more and more frequent. On the day we interviewed him, he had examined a civil servant whose blood sugar was twice the normal level and who also had very high blood pressure. Such lifestyle diseases, he said, have become more and more common, even in the outlying villages that are connected to Madang by roads.

However, another scattering of studies and observations does seem to describe a circumstance of serious under-nutrition—one affecting large numbers of Papua New Guineans, whether rural or urban. Under-nutrition, including a lack of energy-dense, protein-rich foods, has apparently been more of a problem for many Papua New Guineans throughout the country than the opposite. Thus, according to a 1996 nationwide household survey, approximately 42 percent of all Papua New Guineans did not meet the target food-energy requirement of two thousand calories, and the proportion of children with stunted growth and of adults with a body mass index below 18.5 was about twice as high in rural households as in urban households. The differences between rural and urban households did not reflect the number of calories available but the kinds of food available. Rural calories tended to come from foods such as local root crops that are low in energy density, low in protein content, and relatively hard to digest, especially for children. A 1999 Salvation Army Study of the rural Eastern Highlands found that "most people ate a meal only twice a day and sweet potatoes and greens made up the bulk of the diet. Animal protein, usually in small amounts, was included in the diet of families only 6 times per month on an average. The most commonly mentioned animal protein was lamb flaps (48%)."[23] Urban calories tended to come from a range of imported, often processed, and easily digested foods that are as much as 50 percent higher in energy density and protein content.[24] But if being poor in the countryside has big nutritional drawbacks, residents of peri-urban settlements (like Sisiak) are also described as seriously vulnerable to undernourishment: "over 90% of food is purchased at the store or market and often this permits one meal, in the evening."[25]

Clearly, for Joseph, the nutritional threat was that of under- rather than over-nourishment. We doubt that he and the nine other members of his household consumed the national average of 3.4 kg of flaps per person. Not only were Joseph and most of his Sisiak neighbors limited in their capacity to join their more affluent countrymen in choosing an animal protein—including flaps—for an evening meal at home; they were also limited in their capacity to join them in choosing among the offerings for an in-town lunch at a snack bar (locally known as a *kai*— literally, "food"—bar).

Set in high-traffic areas, snack bars are important features of contemporary urban life in Papua New Guinea. Some are lodged inside supermarkets; many are in small shops or open directly onto the street. Most have at least six aluminum food warmers set within glass-fronted, hot-food cabinets so that prospective patrons can readily see the offerings. These are likely to be roasted chicken parts; boiled (or sometimes deep-fried!) lamb flaps; boiled sausages; deep-fried, battered barracuda; chicken or lamb stew; deep-fried flour balls; and French fries. Rice and sometimes boiled plantains with greens or deep-fried sweet potatoes are usual accompaniments. Less frequently offered are lamb hearts, pig trotters, pig jowls, and (formerly) lamb tongues.[26] There are also Cokes and other soft drinks for sale. A meal, which can either be taken away or eaten at a nearby table, is likely to cost at least K3–5 (US$1.00–1.66). At this price, these modernist, energy-dense (and greasily aromatic) foods can be enjoyed only by those with more ready cash than someone like Joseph.

Flaps are also often available at open-air markets, including informal ones along highways. Sold there in bite-sized portions known as *wan maus*—literally, "one mouthful"—they are an affordable luxury even for Joseph. In the Highlands, where flaps are especially popular, we talked to those who cook and sell such portions. In both Mount Hagen and Goroka we watched them—usually women—gathered around a freezer in a local supermarket, choosing the day's flaps. For their selection, cardboard cartons of several brands (each measuring about 55×40×18 cm) had been bandsawed into quarters and halves. Appraising the contents from the sliced-open profiles, customers selected the quarter or half that best met their criteria of value. Prices did vary somewhat, according to the ratio of bone, fat, and meat. (Typically, a quarter-carton weighed 5 kg and cost about K26 [US$8.66]; a half, 10 kg and cost about K50 [US$16.66]). One woman said that she was "tired" of bony flaps, as they were a dead loss. No one would pay 20 toea [about US$.07] for a bony *wan maus*. Another woman said that she chooses flaps that are about half meat and half fat because that is how Highlanders like their flap snacks. Once their selections had been made, payment might be deferred, sometimes until after the day's sales. This was more likely to be the case in smaller stores where a personal relationship with the proprietor existed. Then women would carry their purchases to the market where,

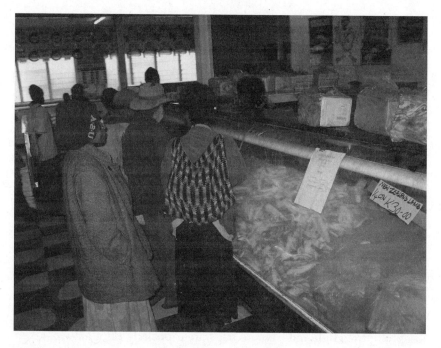

Figure 6. Waiting to buy flaps at a store in Goroka

sometimes with the help of their husbands, they would chop the flaps with a bush knife (machete) into bite-sized portions to be cooked and sold.

All used a cooking apparatus that was simple and portable, usually consisting of an oblong, twenty-liter can (one, for instance, in which a snack bar might have purchased cooking oil) that had been cut open at the sides. When placed on the ground, it could shelter a fire inside and support a metal plate on top (often the lid of a two-hundred-liter fuel drum), on which the pieces, generously salted, sizzled in a fragrant mixture of oil and their own fat. Most vendors simply offered pieces of several sizes, ranging in price from 20 to 50 toea (about US$.07–.17). Some would diversify the menu with sausage pieces. Others would provide slightly fancier and pricier fare. For 50 toea to K1 (US$.17–.33), customers could buy a skewer of flap portions, vegetables, and a ginger slice. As

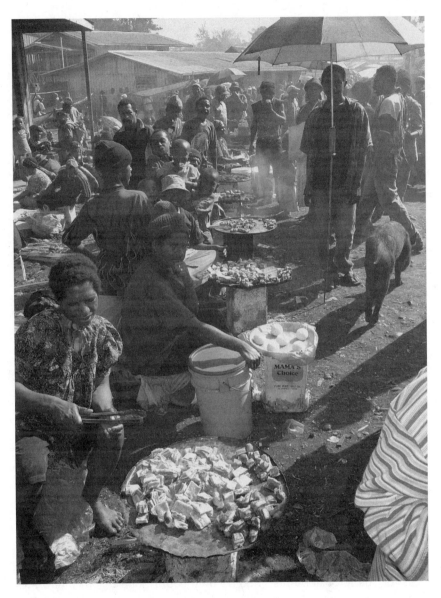

Figure 7. Selling flap pieces at a market in Goroka

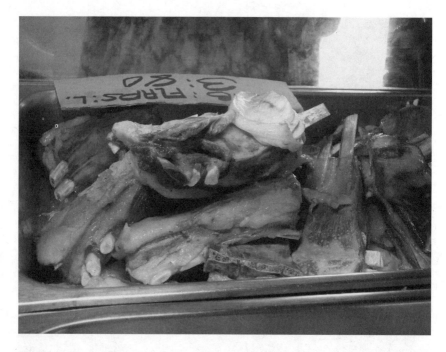

Figure 8.   Cooked flaps for sale at a snack bar in Madang

people shopped, meandered, socialized, or took a break from a dart game, they would stop by the section of the market where the vendors congregated. Once their choice was made, the vendor would pick up the piece with tongs and place it on a scrap of banana leaf—a savory and sustaining flap pick-me-up. (Fred attests that the several salty, fatty, meaty mouthfuls he ate were quite tasty.)

The sellers said that this was their primary source of income and that they made a profit of about K10–15 per day (US$3.33–5.00) when selling quarter-cartons. There was no waste involved—any leftovers were brought home for family consumption. They thought it was a pretty good business for them, or about as good as they could hope for. In interviews with our research assistants, market sellers were unanimous in their opposition to efforts currently afoot to control the sale of flaps. They were aghast to learn that certain Pacific Island nations were considering banning them entirely. Although some sellers admitted that they were dubious about the healthfulness of flaps, none thought they should be banned: what would poor people do to earn money; what would poor people do for food?

When we returned to Madang, we talked to the Papua New Guinea owner and manager of a local snack bar about what we had learned from and about these Highland market sellers. Though her own enterprise was well established, and her clientele were likely to be more affluent than those eating at the market, she too said that she would worry about her business and about feeding the poor if Papua New Guinea were to ban lamb flaps. She herself sold five cartons (100 kg) of lamb and mutton flaps each week. Indeed, she believed that she probably would not have a business if she did not sell flaps. Yet she was ambivalent about them, acknowledging that they are "waste-products being sold to us."

She is not the only Papua New Guinean who has come to feel ambivalent or think critically about flaps. Now that the optimism of the 1970s and 1980s has diminished, she and other Papua New Guineans are realizing that they have to settle for (or indeed, often actively accept) what other people do not want. As we shall see, this conversion of trash into treasure may become, over time, an increasingly compromised alchemy.

FIVE Smiles and Shrugs, Worried Eyes and Sighs

The ambivalence of the Madang snack bar owner concerning lamb and mutton flaps was echoed by many Papua New Guineans, especially by those better able than Joseph to eat their fair share, and more, of the country's flap imports. We first encountered this ambivalence during our preliminary research in 2004. At that time we mentioned to a range of people—mostly with at least a modest income—that we were interested in studying the role of lamb and mutton flaps in Papua New Guinea. Many acquaintances—businessmen, civil servants, teachers, health workers, plantation employees, rural smallholders, market vendors, security guards, storekeepers, shop clerks, hotel staff, and plantation workers—responded in a way that intrigued us. They smiled, but they also shrugged. The smiles, we surmised, signaled recognition that Papua New Guineans do like their flaps; the shrugs, some discomfort from that fact. But all of this would need to be investigated. Our early impressions were, of course, not enough.

We certainly needed to know more about the smiles—more about who ate flaps, how often, and on what occasions. We wished to learn more about consumption not only in such contexts as urban snacking and family eating, but also during collective events. These would include the church functions we had attended at Ramu Sugar, Limited (RSL) and also the "traditional" exchanges for which Papua New Guinea has become famous. If, as we had been told by colleagues, flaps were increasingly important in ceremonial life, what did this indicate?[1] Various possibilities came to mind. Perhaps the most interesting was that flaps might be displacing pigs, which (alive, cooked, or raw) had been a crucial component of many ritual exchanges, especially in the Highlands. What, then, would it mean if a creature nurtured by family members, fed from the family gardens, and sheltered in or near the family house was being displaced by an already dead and dismembered foreign product purchased with the cash earned from the sale of commercial crops or labor? The presentation of a family pig, almost a family member itself, had made sense in a circumstance of ongoing reciprocation, of long-term social entailment. What would the presentation of lamb and mutton flaps suggest about contemporary Papua New Guinean social circumstances?

In thinking about how relationships established through pigs might differ from those established through flaps, we reminded ourselves that items that had their origin as commodities could serve well as gifts. Indeed, as we saw in chapter 4, part of the promise of development was its ability to provide the money and goods that would allow village people to arrange bigger and better ceremonies. (And, of course, Western consumers also transform commodities into gifts on ceremonial occasions, such as on birthdays and Christmas, through thoughtful selection, removal of price tags, and careful wrapping.[2]) We would also have to keep in mind that items that had their origins as (potential) gifts could serve well as commodities. Certainly, some people in contemporary Papua New Guinea earn at least part of their income from the sale of their family pigs—often to those who wish to use them in ceremonies. Thus, although we suspected that the substitution of purchased flaps for home-grown pigs at ceremonies marked a transformation, we did not think it represented any simple shift between types of relationships—between the personal and impersonal, the ongoing and sharply circumscribed. Indeed, we were fascinated to find out more about what flaps were helping to make happen.

We also wanted to understand more about the shrugs. If, as we thought, they indicated discomfort, what were its sources? We knew that flaps sometimes receive critical press in Papua New Guinea. Flaps have been singled out, for example, in occasional articles about the connection between fats and lifestyle diseases. One that appeared in the *Reporter* (a university newsletter produced by students at Lae Technical College) listed lamb flaps as a fatty meat and advised that "fat is indeed a major contributor to the incidence of heart disease, cancer, obesity and other chronic diseases."[3] We were particularly interested in a letter in the *National* newspaper arguing that local people's "huge appetite for imported goods" like these meat products had led to an unfortunate food dependence on "foreign-controlled business houses" and that flaps should be banned from the country.[4] Did others share this larger concern that the trade in flaps contributed to the country's postcolonial vulnerability by maintaining its dependence on imports?[5]

Several articles talked not only about health concerns, but also about the connections between such problems and the status of Papua New Guineans in the world. The *Post Courier* cited a physician who had to face "the daily suffering and problems related to diabetes, heart disease, arthritis and other systemic diseases" and who was demanding to know why the health inspectors were not doing more to keep lamb flaps out of Papua New Guinea—"this junk food, which in other countries is processed for dog and cat food."[6] In fact, such concerns are long-standing. In 1996 Daniel Kapi, the executive director of the Papua New Guinea Consumer Affairs Council, protested that "Lamb flaps are not 'meat' . . . in the sense of what . . . [white people] would consider meat." Though not advocating a ban on the import of flaps, he asserted that exporters had "a moral obligation not to dump cheap junk on us" and that they should only send flaps that were "90 per cent meat and 10 percent fat."[7]

We were interested in knowing whether Papua New Guineans knew about such concerns and, if they did, whether flaps had perhaps become so central to Papua New Guinea life that people could not imagine giving them up in any case. A comparison we had in mind was "chitlins"—pigs' intestines, often battered and fried, which have become for some African Americans a repository of history and a validation of ethnic identity.[8] To elicit an overall appraisal of whether Papua New Guineans felt that they would be better off with or without flaps, we wished to know if people thought that their government should ban their importation. We knew that we needed help in our investigation, not only because of what we saw as the complexity of flaps, but also because of what we saw as the complexity of our asking about flaps, which might generate even more ambivalence. What were Papua New Guineans to make of the interest we, as white people—who might be known as generally eschewing this food—had in learning about why they ate so much of it? While anthropologists can, with time, build sufficient trust with local people to converse relatively frankly about potentially touchy issues, including mutual racial and social differences, we could not hope to do so with Papua New Guineans we had never met before.[9]

To help us, therefore, we hired a research team of Papua New Guineans, mostly students at Madang's Divine Word University, who had been trained in research methods by Nancy Sullivan (an anthropologist and long-term resident of Papua New Guinea).[10] Since flaps are sold and eaten primarily in urban areas, where electricity allows them to be frozen or at least refrigerated, we asked the team to administer questionnaires in five towns: the coastal (lowland) towns of Madang and Gusap, and the Highland towns of Goroka, Mount Hagen, and Kerowagi. Our research team stationed themselves near stores, outdoor markets, and bus stops. There they stopped passersby, explaining that they wished to interview them and record the interview on a questionnaire as part of a project on the circulation of lamb and mutton flaps throughout the Pacific Islands. They also gave assurance that anonymity would be preserved.[11]

We did not intend these interviews to be a definitive survey about the role of lamb and mutton flaps throughout the country. We knew that there were Papua New Guineans living in remote locations, including some in the Chambri Lakes, who rarely, if ever, ate flaps. Instead, we sought material that would broadly illustrate the range of practices and perceptions in regard to flaps. We instructed the interviewers not to focus on people they already knew, but to elicit information from a wide variety of individuals. We asked them to describe briefly the appearance and manner of those they interviewed, and to indicate whether any of them were previous acquaintances. In the end, they interviewed an appropriate variety of individuals (only a few of whom had been known to them) and often described their interviewees in a rather detailed manner—distinguishing, for example, between a person who was "well-dressed and well spoken" (i.e., affluent and modern) from someone who was "a typical village person dressed in rags" (i.e., poor and "traditional").

The interviewers began their questions by collecting basic demographic data. They interviewed 146 men and 143 women of a range of ages.[12] They also recorded occupations: 127 received regular salaries or wages (although their incomes, as we shall see, varied considerably); 100 earned money informally or were self-employed (their incomes also varied considerably);[13] and 62 were unemployed.[14]

They then asked informants how often they ate flaps. (The answers varied from not at all to daily.) What brands of flaps did they favor and why? (The answers varied from no preference, to preference for a brand thought to be especially fatty, or relatively lean, or relatively bone-free.) When and where did they and/or others they knew eat flaps? (The answers varied from lunch counters or the market, to family meals, to ceremonial feasts.) What meats, in ceremonial contexts, had been replaced by flaps, to what extent, and why? (The answers varied from just augmentation without replacement because pigs, chickens, and fish remain important, to complete replacement of pigs because pigs are too much work and are prohibited to Seventh-day Adventists.) What health implications did flaps have? (The answers varied from none, to causing a variety of illnesses, including asthma, arthritis, and heart attacks.) And finally, should the government ban flaps from the country? (The answers varied from no, because they are a good, cheap source of protein, or because poor people make money vending them, or because they have become part of Papua New Guinea culture; to yes, because they are health hazards or are waste products that white New Zealanders and Australians will not eat.)

As we sorted through these data, we discovered a set of overlapping themes that we characterize below, illustrating each with a summary of an interview.

Flaps as an Unambiguous Good

This was the view of a thirty-year-old married woman, originally from a village in the Southern Highlands Province, who lives with her husband and three children in a settlement outside of Mount Hagen and supports her family by selling lamb and mutton flaps at the market. She said that she buys a quarter-carton of lamb and mutton flaps every day for sale. She likes to purchase hers from one particular store because it offers the greasiest and meatiest flaps, which appeal to lots of people at the market and provide her with a decent profit. Although pigs are still mandatory at all major ceremonies back in the village, flaps are always suitable nowadays as well. She is very much against the possibility that the government might ban lamb and mutton flaps because they are the only meat that people can afford and, for people like her, the only source of income for the family.

Flaps as a Slightly Ambiguous Good

This was the view of a twenty-four-year-old man, originally from (coastal) East New Britain Province, who lives with his wife's family in a settlement outside of Goroka, works as a store clerk, and earns K70 a fortnight (US$23). He said that he supplements his income by cooking and vending bite-sized portions of lamb and mutton flaps at the market, buying about four cartons a week.[15] He'll buy a quarter- or half-carton at a time. The business is lucrative, especially on the weekends, when there are lots of drunk people around who enjoy a snack. There are many people like him who buy flaps to sell at the market, at the side of the road, or at mini-shops. But it is common for people to buy cartons to feed those attending a party—for example, after a sporting event, for a business opening, or during a political campaign. Lamb and mutton flaps are also often served at church events or as part of customary occasions such as wedding celebrations, mortuary rituals, and compensation payments. In the Highlands, pigs remain the most valued food for most customary occasions (his particular community favors fish), but more and more people are substituting lamb and mutton flaps because they taste good and are affordable. It is true that lamb and mutton flaps are very fatty, but most people do not care about this since the meat is cheap and delicious. They have become a normal part of major ceremonies. Therefore, the government should not ban them.

Flaps as Cheap and Convenient, If Possibly Unhealthy

This was the view of a thirty-seven-year-old married woman, originally from Goroka, who lives at Gusap (where her husband works for Ramu Sugar, earning about K700 a fortnight [US$233]) and who occasionally sells peanuts at the market to supplement the family income. She said that she buys flaps about two times a week in 2 kg packages to feed her husband and five children. They like them best when mixed with greens and rice. Sometimes, when she has to contribute to a funeral or compensation ceremony, she will buy flaps in a carton. Although pigs and chickens remain people's favorites, flaps are making their way into ceremonies because they are cheap and go a long way to feed many people. Also, many people cannot take care of pigs because they have other things to do. The government would be crazy to ban flaps. If they are really not safe for human consumption, the government must provide an alternative source of protein at a reduced price.

Flaps as Cheap, Tasty, and "Ours," but No Substitute for Pigs

This was the view of a forty-four-year-old married man, born in a village near Mount Hagen, who lives in a settlement within the town and supports himself by selling betel nuts at the market. He said that he buys lamb and mutton flaps in bite-sized pieces all the time at the market and in quarter-cartons occasionally to feed his family. He thinks flaps from Australia are the best because they are the biggest ones available. Although pigs remain the most important item of exchange at weddings, compensations, and other ceremonies, some people contribute flaps to these occasions. Lamb and mutton flaps are OK, but some will think that those who only bring flaps to ceremonies are pretenders who cut corners. Killing a pig shows that you have respect for your guests and, if you kill one, people will look at you as a real "big man." He himself will buy a pig from those who raise them with the money he earns through his betel nut sales. From his perspective, the government should not ban flaps. They are good meat for the "grassroots" (poor people). Most everything else is too expensive, and Papua New Guineans have gotten used to flaps. They are part of Papua New Guinea.

Flaps as Tasty and Cheap, but an Inferior Food

This is the view of a forty-five-year-old man, originally from the Southern Highlands town of Tari, who lives at Gusap and works as a seasonal employee at Ramu Sugar, earning (when he works) K150 a fortnight (US$50). He said that he buys flaps whenever he feels the desire for them, maybe once a fortnight while he is working for money. He likes meaty lamb and mutton flaps the best and finds them the most savory. Although pigs are still important, flaps have become acceptable at many ceremonies, such as funerals, weddings, and church celebrations. They are also distributed during political campaigns when politicians want people to vote for them. They are used because they feed a lot of people inexpensively. Although he enjoys them, especially when they are mixed with greens in a soup, he has heard that they are not good—that white men do not eat them, but feed them to their dogs and other animals. Papua New Guineans should not eat food that is bad for them and so, if the government decides to ban them, he will support the decision.

Flaps as Useful, If Low-Quality, but Dumped on Papua New Guinea

This is the view of a thirty-two-year-old, married man, originally from a coastal area of the Morobe Province, who lives in a settlement near the Goroka Secondary School and works as a security guard, earning K120 a fortnight (US$40). He said that he buys flaps in small packages about three times a week. He has attended reconciliation ceremonies where flaps were cooked and then exchanged between the feuding parties. He also buys cartons for birthday celebrations. He knows that in the past pigs, as symbols of hard work and big-manship, would be brought to all ceremonies. Lamb and mutton flaps are rapidly replacing them in importance because they are easier to get. Though some object to their greasiness, he likes them, believing that they have helped him become big and strong. Yet he grants that many people are dying because flaps cause heart disease and asthma. He thinks that they should be banned because New Zealand and Australia are dumping them in Papua New Guinea. Papua New Guinea should only accept quality meat from these places.

Flaps as Useful and Cheap, but Unhealthful, Making People Lazy, and Dumped on Papua New Guinea

This is the view of a twenty-seven-year-old, unmarried woman, originally from the Central Province, who lives on the campus of the Goroka school at which she teaches, earning K300 a fortnight (US$100). She said that she buys small packages of lamb and mutton flaps about once a week, preferring those from one of two stores because they are tender and less greasy than the others. Since she never buys them in cartons, she is not sure where they come from, but she thinks most come from New Zealand. She chooses flaps that have the rib bones showing because these have more meat than fat. She knows many people living in settlements and villages throughout the Highlands who buy cartons of flaps for bride-price payments, death ceremonies, and other customary events. Lamb and mutton flaps are popular for these purposes because they are the cheapest meat an ordinary Papua New Guinean can acquire. She is in favor of a ban on lamb and mutton flaps, however, because their availability has made people lazy about raising other forms of protein, like pigs. Also, lamb and mutton flaps are unhealthy and reduce the lifespan of the people. Papua New Guinea should not be a rubbish dump.

*Flaps as Useful and Cheap, but Unhealthy and a Drain
on the Papua New Guinean Economy*

This is the view of a twenty-nine-year-old coffee-grower who lives with his wife and three children in a village some distance from Mount Hagen and had come to town on some "personal" business. He said that he buys flaps in small quantities for family consumption from time to time, choosing the meatiest and least greasy ones because he is worried about high blood-pressure and heart disease. He has also contributed flaps to bride-price payments and to compensate fellow villagers who help him with his coffee trees. Although people would still prefer to give pigs, they are too expensive. Lamb and mutton flaps are cheap and can be bought in large quantities to feed many people. Nonetheless, he would like them banned because they take money out of the country. However, to ban them would mean that the government must find a cheap substitute for them.

·   ·   ·   ·   ·

In the corpus of the interviews (as well as the individual ones cited above), we found that most Papua New Guineans generally accept lamb and mutton flaps as useful, albeit with reservations. Of course, some like them more than others. Some like their greasy taste, or the greasy flavor they give to carbohydrates and greens, while others do not. Some believe that they are strengthened by flaps, others that they are sickened— mentioning ailments ranging from heart attacks to (the more medically dubious) asthma, arthritis, and even, in several interviews, sagging skin. However, virtually all Papua New Guineans will eat flaps if they can get them. (In fact, one Papua New Guinean physician told us that because flaps are cheap and tasty and his hospital salary is not large, he and his family eat more flaps than he knows they should—this despite the fact that two of his colleagues died from heart disease.)

If flaps do not provide Papua New Guineans with the food they need to survive under difficult financial circumstances, they do provide many with an occasional taste treat. In addition, there is ample evidence that lamb and mutton flaps have become increasingly important, often central, in constructing various forms of social relationships through exchange. Many urban-dwelling Papua New Guineans in our sample wish to nurture relationships with kinsmen in their villages of origin—not least of all because they suspect that they may have to return to these villages when they retire or when the cash demands of urban life become overwhelming. To nurture these relationships, they must contribute to important life-cycle ceremonies, such as weddings and funerals, and to redressive ceremonies, like compensations for injuries or deaths. To this end, they often use flaps. However, most Papua New Guineans in our sample, as well as those we talked to ourselves, agreed that, regardless of whether flaps are offered, a major ceremony *must* have at least one pig. This is true not only for the Highlanders (who, in fact, would find a ceremony with only a single pig inadequate) but also, we venture, for most Papua New Guineans. It is certainly true for Chambri, who stressed that a life-cycle ceremony must feature a pig whose killing marks the transition.

Part of the significance of pigs is that, under village circumstances, a great deal of labor goes into raising them.[16] Pigs have to be sheltered, restrained, and fed. (In one classic study of a Highland community, the anthropologist Roy Rappaport calculated that 13–15 pigs kept by four households over an eight-month period "received considerably more sweet potato and manioc than did the 16 humans. . . . 53.7% of the total" garden crop brought to houses.[17]) Compromises may, however, be made. One Papua New Guinean businessman in Goroka told us that he has no time to raise pigs himself but keeps six penned on his village land under the care of his kinsmen, so that they are available when needed. It is also common to buy a pig, provided one has the money—K700 [US$233] and upwards. This is what the betel nut seller from Mount Hagen advocated in order to avoid being regarded as a pretender to big-man status by people back home. Many urban dwellers, however, do not have the money to buy pigs, and most lack the time and inclination to raise them. Some went so far as to say that those who raise pigs are "wasting their time" and "have nothing better to do." Therefore, to meet their ceremonial obligations in an acceptable, if not stellar, manner, they purchase lamb and mutton flaps.

A Goroka-based Papua New Guinean importer and purveyor of flaps explained the huge demand for lamb and mutton flaps for use in ceremonies as due in part to the growing popularity throughout the country of Seventh-day Adventism (a religion that prohibits the consumption of pork) as well as to the fact that those who work for money simply find raising pigs not worth the time and trouble involved.[18] Instead of contributing pigs to a ceremony, they will contribute between two and ten cartons of flaps (perhaps augmented with a purchased pig), since flaps presented in multiple cartons can appear reasonably impressive and are readily matched to the occasion. Those giving them will say, " 'This is our contribution; this is our thank you for looking after things here; we trust you are happy.' And then people eat together and everyone can go around free [from recrimination]—including back to town."

In effect, there is a continuum on which homegrown pigs, purchased pigs, and flaps are located. The heaviest and most intractable obligations are responded to with pigs; the lightest and most flexible, with flaps. Flaps are the professions and facilitators of an ongoing affability, one consistent with commensality; they mark and foster relationships of goodwill among kin who no longer engage with one another frequently. Such was the case with a family group we heard discussing plans to buy flaps for a visiting relative's send-off feast; they were deciding whether they might be able to spring for a full carton, rather than a half (and whether either one would place an undue burden on the relative when the time came for this person to reciprocate). Flaps also mark and foster relationships of goodwill between colleagues, teammates, and neighbors who are well-disposed but have few long-term commitments to one another. Flaps are, in other words, both convenient and sufficient, and as such they allow urban dwellers with some money to maintain ties to village kin as well as to extend relationships to urban friends.

As edible tokens of ongoing and shifting commitments, lamb and mutton flaps are useful in their capacity to be used flexibly. In this regard, Papua New Guineans are adding value to flaps, in that flaps allow for the creation of ties that variously bind—and do not bind. However, to take flaps, which have become widely understood as another's rejects, and use them for one's own purposes remains, for many—at least for the present—a compromised practice. Thus, as our interview data indicate, Papua New Guineans do know—and do remain concerned by the fact— that lamb and mutton flaps are rejected by white people. This, we think, leads to a diffuse social anxiety that may be reflected in the diffuse range of maladies attributed to flaps. Consequently, Papua New Guineans some-times worry that their bodies, identities, and social relationships depend on "treasuring" what they know to be other people's "trash." Perhaps this accounts for the smiles and shrugs we mentioned earlier.

WORRIED EYES AND SIGHS

To be unable to realize a compromised practice moves many Papua New Guineans from ambivalence to distress: to eat what white people eschew is a problem; to be unable to afford what white people eschew is a bigger problem. This is true for people like Joseph and even more so for those at Ramu Sugar, whose expectations are much higher. What for some are smiles and shrugs, for them become worried eyes and sighs.

We had, as mentioned, already spent considerable time at RSL. A Papua New Guinean agro-industrial sugar complex, RSL was built in the early 1980s as a centerpiece of development in a newly independent nation. It was to be a place of work where Papua New Guinean employ-ees from all over the country would learn the modern technical skills and disciplines necessary to grow, process, and package sugar. It was also to be a place of residence where employees would enjoy with their nuclear families the rewards of their hard-won modernity. With reason-able salaries and with housing and utilities provided, they would lead pleasant, amenity-filled lives—including access to churches, schools, health clinics, and the small commercial center of Gusap. We came to respect, if not to admire, much about RSL. However, the hard times the country was going through were also adversely affecting the company's fortunes and the lives of most of its Papua New Guinean employees. There was not enough money to enable these employees, even those well-educated ones in top managerial positions (who had passed all exams from standard six through university), to afford much of the promise of a developed life.

On numerous occasions during the course of our RSL research, we had met with one such well-educated manager, Marcus Nembwi (a pseudonym), who worked in RSL's agricultural division earning approximately K900/fortnight (US$300). (We had an immediate bond because he was a friend of a young Chambri man whose education Deborah had helped finance.) Born in 1965 in the town of Wewak, where his father was the gardener for the Catholic Bishop, he and his family eventually moved back to their home village. There he was educated at schools run by the Assemblies of God mission, where he was taught "honesty, righteousness, living straight, and respecting others as yourself." Passing all of his exams, he won a place at Karavat National High School, which was located in the "advanced agricultural province" of East New Britain. Thus he became interested in agricultural science and attended the University of Papua New Guinea. He was a good student and won a scholarship in 1984 to study in Japan, but he stayed just six months because he was "only nineteen and put alone into the heart of a big city." Although he had been confident at home that he could do anything, in Japan he lost his confidence and became homesick. So he returned to Papua New Guinea and finished his tertiary degree at Lae Technical College. After working at various positions (including with a mining company for which he did environmental research), he took a job at RSL—hired first in a supervisory position but soon promoted to a managerial one. At RSL he was active in his Four Square church, contributing significantly with labor and materials to the construction of a pastor's house and four school classrooms. He and his wife have limited their family size. Many Papua New Guineans, he said, believe that lots of children will provide them with "security and with flexibility in their old age—the ability to move from one child's house to another." But he does not want such dependence. He also thinks it would be just too expensive to feed and school many children.

As it is, he feels short of money—and this is so even though his wife works as well (as a secretary at RSL). Like most families at RSL, his is forced to "cut down on meat because protein is expensive." Lamb flaps are cheap—at the two mini-supermarkets from which RSL employees purchase food, they were selling during our 2006 research at about K8.50/kg (US$2.83)—and they blend well with rice and greens. All can be boiled up together with coconut cream. Yet even flaps are not cheap enough to have very frequently; in fact, because of the cost of meat, he and his family have almost become vegetarians. They buy lamb and mutton flaps maybe once in a fortnight, on payday, and at other times scatter bits of canned tuna on their vegetables or, as a real indulgence, purchase a live chicken. At least he does not have the anxiety of chronic debt; he knows many workers who week after week have to borrow money at loan-shark rates against the next paycheck.[19] But given his hard work and education, he is somewhat dissatisfied with the life he leads. He hopes eventually to "follow his dream": to work with donor agencies interested in helping farmers form cooperatives, manage fields, and acquire credit.

Marcus's circumstances were consistent with those suggested by the data collected for us by another RSL employee. Philip Klomes interviewed twenty-two of his co-workers, ranging in grade from 2 to 12 (and earning salaries from K125.45 to K900/fortnight [US$41.84–US$300]), concerning their "shopping baskets." According to his survey, all buy virtually the same items every two weeks, though in varying amounts depending on their salaries and family size. In addition to the nonfood essentials (soap, bleach, razor blades, deodorant or perfume), the basics are rice, sugar, cooking oil, canned fish, instant noodles, and local vegetables from the open-air market. The desirable, if limited, supplements are chicken wings, chicken tails, pig tails (or another cheap cut of pork, like jowls or trotters), lamb and mutton flaps, and canned corned beef. A live chicken, purchased rarely, is an extravagance. Philip included an essay of explanation with the data, in which he concluded that many workers are "sacrificing themselves to budget for the school fees of their children, which are given first priority" and therefore cannot afford much store-bought food. "The major protein eaten by most employees in Ramu is Diana tuna," he wrote, "and some can afford the K1.40 for a small can [US$.47 for 185 g] only every 2–3 days." He himself found this conclusion rather disturbing, and he commented that, given his salary of K232.22 (US$77.41) and four children to support, he wondered about his own financial situation. He had hoped his job at RSL would lead to a "better life," but instead life was a "constant struggle." He was doing his best by taking correspondence courses, but these were expensive. He hoped we might help arrange a scholarship for him, or perhaps help him acquire a used laptop computer.

There were others connected to RSL who had begun to enjoy at least some of the promises of modernity only to find them slipping away. Mari villagers living in the vicinity of the plantation had, until recently, been earning a regular income from RSL for sugarcane grown on their land. They were the envy of many other Papua New Guineans, for whom cash (and, as we have seen, sometimes food) was often short. They had enough money to cover school fees, to buy commodities such as sneakers and bicycles (and sometimes even television sets and generators), and to drink beer, play snooker, and splurge on ritual occasions. The regular income also allowed them considerable choice in their diets. They could easily supplement their garden produce with store-bought food, which frequently included lamb and mutton flaps. One Mari friend told us of his enjoyment of every aspect of the flap experience—from walking out of a Gusap mini-supermarket with a hefty bag of frozen flaps in each hand, to the anticipation of the meal, to licking up the grease that oozed from the corners of his mouth when the meal was over.

These resources allowed particular Mari and their families not only to enjoy the good life, but also to create contexts of inclusive and mutually affirming sociality. Families contributed quantities of food for general consumption at church picnics, and ritual events such as funerals provided opportunities for even more lavish generosity. After the sudden death of the highly respected RSL manager responsible for dealing with the Mari landowners, for example, the Mari were able to contribute large amounts of food, including lamb and mutton flaps, to feed the hundreds of mourners. Though clearly upset by the death, they took satisfaction from responding impressively and appropriately. Their affluence allowed them a public generosity that presented them at their best.

However, in 2003 the situation changed. Several ethnic groups living in the region had long been challenging Mari claims upon the land.

Eventually, under court order, RSL was forced to place the payments for the sugar grown on this land into an escrow account until the rightful owners could be determined. Although some Mari found seasonal or low-level jobs at RSL, their income, along with their standard of living and standing in the world, was drastically diminished. Payment of school fees, especially for children who had gone beyond the relatively inexpensive lower grades of the village school, became a real problem. Some academically qualified children were held back to cycle again through the village school; some who were already in the upper grades were withdrawn from school altogether. Shopping for store-bought food was greatly reduced, and luxury goods were all sold. Even the possibility of a favorable court outcome was somewhat compromised, as Mari had accumulated considerable debt to pay their lawyers by borrowing against a future win in court.[20] They had, for the time at least, become just another "grassroots" group scraping by.

When we last spoke with them during 2006, their earlier life of affluence, including their consumption of lamb and mutton flaps, had become a thing of the past. As of this writing, the legal case, after numerous delays, is still unresolved.[21]

BEING FAT IN PAPUA NEW GUINEA

When we met with Dr. Mosey Sau, the physician at RSL, he told us that relatively few of his patients suffered from lifestyle diseases associated with over-nutrition—hypertension, diabetes, and myocardial infarction. He was not surprised, since RSL's population was both young and physically active. There were few employees older than fifty, and most worked quite hard. Hypertension was most likely to afflict employees for whom the stresses of factory work were difficult to manage. (When visiting the factory, we had wondered how workers, during the long harvest season shifts, coped with the heat, noise, and steam while monitoring and adjusting the industrial processes by which cane became sugar.) Adult onset diabetes was most prevalent among employees who had lived in urban areas.

When we asked him about lamb and mutton flaps as contributors to such diseases, he doubted that, even if eaten once or twice a week, they would be particularly harmful. Given that most employees burn a lot of calories while working, he thought that fatty meats might actually be good for them, since fat, as we have seen, is needed to process fat-soluble vitamins.

But what of fat Papua New Guineans? We asked several Mari what they thought of fat people. Paul Emmanuel, one of our research assistants, provided a typical answer. He said that he was sorry for them because they could work for only about thirty minutes before they ran out of breath, became sweaty, and had to stop and rest. They could not climb mountains. They were slow. And, Paul joked, if their enemies came, they could not flee. Indeed, most Mari found the bulk of those few Mari who were fat rather amusing, a source of good-natured banter. For example, Paul often joshed with one, telling him, for instance, that now that he could no longer afford flaps, he was getting the exercise he needed—trudging through the cane fields to catch fish at the river. Others may feel similarly amused, to judge by an item in the news-about-town feature in the *Post Courier,* which reported that during a recent "downpour, passengers in a bus swinging around the huge Koki market roundabout were stunned to see a huge guy, lamb flaps hanging over his waist and at both sides, bare-chested, trying to shelter under the denuded trees in the middle of the roundabout. . . . He nonchalantly saluted the passengers with his ice-cream cone. All burst into laughter at the sight."[22]

Most RSL employees and Mari—and, we venture, many *Post Courier* readers—would view eating lamb and mutton flaps at home, at a snack bar, at the market, or at a ceremony as an appropriate and reasonable expression of their aspirations. If such people became fat because they ate too many flaps, they might be met with amusement but not condemnation. However, if members of the elite overindulged, they would likely get a quite different response.

Indeed, many were appalled by the corpulence of national politicians—who, together with civil servants, are most responsible for the rise in the number of cardiovascular patients admitted to Port Moresby General Hospital.[23] Many ordinary Papua New Guineans whom we know regard

the corpulence of politicians as the most salient mark of class differences.[24] Thus when non-elite Papua New Guineans said, as they often did,
that their politicians looked "pregnant with twins," they were comment-
ing not only on their appearance but on their corruption. They were making a wry, cynical, and anxious comment about a disordered world in
which the bulk of politicians is an index of their illegitimate and disproportionate power and privilege. These men—or at least some of them—
travel all over the world at public expense and have amassed enough
money to educate their children in Australia and New Zealand and to buy
Australian property in Cairns and on the Gold Coast. They not only
have access to all of the lamb and mutton flaps they may or may not wish
to eat but are notorious for regularly enjoying steaks and beer (and
women) at hotels. As one young Mari man told us, when he sees a fat politician, he is afraid. He knows that this man, with his obvious resources
and connections, can eat anything he desires and do virtually anything he
wants. He knows that if there were a reason to take a politician or another
comparably rich man to court, there would be little point in doing so. Unfortunately, rich people, virtually all Papua New Guineans agree, almost
always win.

THE GOOD LIFE?

We have argued that the Pacific Island trade in lamb and mutton flaps
links and distinguishes broad categories of people. We have met representatives of two of these categories: those who provide, trade, and for the
most part eschew flaps; and those who buy and eat them, though sometimes with ambivalence. We have also seen that this trade is no simple
manifestation of the free-market truth that meat never goes uneaten. Even
if the price is right, the traffic in cheap, fatty meat is likely to be politically
charged.

Among those least willing to regard the purchase and consumption
of flaps as simply the neutral outcomes of the market are those who
strongly associate flaps with lifestyle diseases and with the unfortunate
economic dependencies of Third World nations. While we are sympa-

thetic to their perspective, we think it has its limitations with respect to the lives of the many undernourished Papua New Guineans still influenced by the elusive promise of development. Should Joseph, for example, be encouraged to return to his subsistence-level and sorcery-afflicted home village to contend with his local adversaries rather than struggle to raise his family at Sisiak? And should Highland women be encouraged to return to their remote villages to raise pigs rather than stay in town to sell flaps at the market?

Indeed, many Papua New Guineans regard flaps as denoting about as much of the good life as will come their way. Certainly, for urban dwellers, flaps are cheap, flavorful protein that feeds their families and provides some with a small income. As these people often told us, if the government plans to ban flaps, it must first find a protein substitute that poor people can afford. For the Mari, flaps once enabled them to feel that they could enjoy the modern good life, both as individuals and as members of social networks. For plantation workers, they remain a suitable, if occasional, reward for their paid employment—their regimented work in a nontraditional, industrial setting. And for those, like Joseph, who are seriously short of cash, flaps represent what life should be like. These Papua New Guineans, thus, would like to have flaps as a modernist staple.[25] Nevertheless, flap eaters often know that they are eating and enjoying the waste products of white people—what white people feed to their dogs. As we have seen, this makes their identity as flap eaters troubling.

However, those whose identity is especially troubling—as least in the eyes of the flap eaters—are the more voracious Papua New Guinean elite who "look pregnant with twins." They can eat whatever they choose, whenever and wherever they want. They are the postcolonial powerful— the First Worlders within—whose lives, resources, and goals are different from those of the rest of their countrymen. Part of what is especially troubling, we think, is that such people are voluntarily rejecting what for other Papua New Guineans is becoming (at least in aspiration) a staple. Staples constitute and define what people regard as the minimal conditions of existence. As such, they have both prescriptive and proscriptive implications. To find staples unaffordable means that one is deprived of something that is almost a right. To be able to afford staples means that one can live an appropriate, although not greatly embellished, life. Yet, to go so far as to reject staples for something deemed better (perhaps to consider staples not as proper food at all) is to exempt oneself from the constraints and standards by which others live.

Hence, what it means to belong to any of the disparate (totemic) groups created and marked by the flow of this cheap, fatty meat is not just a neutral outcome of an impartial market that allocates goods according to supply and demand. It is also an outcome of the broader system of discontinuous differences through which lamb and mutton flaps (and those who do or do not eat them) are evaluated. As we have said, the transformation of trash to treasure is a compromised alchemy.

SIX Pacific Island Flaps

The Papua New Guineans who were seeking to curtail the trade in flaps did not have much effect.[1] However, their counterparts elsewhere in the Pacific have been somewhat more successful. At about the same time that Papua New Guinea's Daniel Kapi was calling for the regulation of lamb and mutton flaps in 1996, other influential Pacific Islanders were expressing similar concerns in public statements. In both Fiji and Tonga, their concerns led to efforts to restrict, if not ban, their sale. Although little was actually enacted in Tonga (for reasons we shall explore), in 2000 Fiji did enact such a ban. The measure was and still is controversial because it challenges the neoliberal market ideology and free-trade practices endorsed by the World Trade Organization (WTO), which allow only a limited regulatory role for governments. Governments are expected to step in, for example, to ensure that appropriate standards of food purity are met, but decisions about whether or not to buy lamb and mutton flaps should be left to consumers.

Such an ideology, of course, exacerbates the global omnivore's dilemma of what to choose to eat. But at least in the case of flaps, it could be argued that what is offered for choice can be appraised clearly. Flaps have no dirty stories pertaining to either their production or their composition. They reveal themselves to consumers as exactly what they are: very fatty meat. Under these circumstances, should people be protected from choosing them? While there may be general agreement that a government should circumscribe market availability of certain addictive ingestibles (e.g., heroin, or tobacco and alcohol for minors),[2] flaps (whatever their appeal and their effects) clearly appear to be a different sort of substance. Given all of this, would it be legitimate for a government to intervene in the trade in flaps beyond, at most, informing citizens about healthful eating?

These considerations focus on issues of broad significance concerning how life should be managed and by whom. What or who should be responsible for determining how risk—whether to individuals, to groups, or to the society itself—is determined and regulated? What are the limits of public health and public interest? If the 290-pound Tongan woman we read about wants to eat 2 kg of lamb and mutton flaps a day, whose business is it? Who should determine whether this woman knows enough about the ramifications of her choices? What of the King of Tonga, the world's most enormous monarch, who in many ways was the primary representative of his people? Who should regulate him? And, closer to home, consider a recent *New York Times* report (July 22, 2007). It describes certain offerings at Burger King, such as "the BK Stacker with four beef patties, and an Enormous Omelet sandwich, which is a sausage, bacon and cheese omelet on a bun. . . . [or] its Meat 'Normous, a breakfast sandwich that the company pitches with this slogan: 'A full pound of sausage, bacon and ham. Have a meaty morning.'"[3] Who is to stop one from having such a morning?

Here we focus on the ways these questions have been addressed in Fiji and Tonga. In the conclusion, we discuss the ways they have been framed in the United States and applied to Tonga and other Pacific Islands.

ON THE HEALTH OF FIJIANS

Our focus on lamb and mutton flaps led us from Papua New Guinea to Fiji, primarily because Fiji has banned the sale of flaps since 2000. We wished to explore the contrast between Papua New Guinea and Fiji. During relatively brief trips to the capital city of Suva in 2004 and 2006, we explored the ban with health professionals, government officials, and ordinary people. We explained that our project was comparative—that we were interested in the different ways that Pacific Island nations sought to protect the health of their citizens. The response we often heard was that Fiji had not only a far more serious problem with lifestyle diseases than did Papua New Guinea, but also a government more committed to and more capable of addressing that problem. Even though the Fijian economy is vulnerable (especially given declines in the sugar and textile industries), and the government is prone to coups, the country is more developed and better organized. This was also the perception of New Zealand and Australian traders, who had told us that they could sell a wider range of products in Fiji, enjoy accommodations of an international standard, and feel safe most of the time.

Fijian health professionals start with certain fundamental observations about their country. The population (some nine hundred thousand in 2007) is divided almost equally between indigenous Fijians and Indo-Fijians, many of whom are descendants of indentured Indians who, as part of the circulation of labor within the British Empire, were brought to Fiji between 1879 and 1916 to work in the sugarcane industry. Until the 1990s, Indo-Fijians were more at risk for cardiovascular disease than the indigenous Fijians. However, since that time, the indigenous Fijians—especially the bureaucrats, for whom relative prosperity has meant butter for breakfast, sausages for lunch, and flaps or some other fatty food for dinner—have become increasingly ill.

The majority of Fijians, living as they do along the coast of the country's largest island, Viti Levu, have relatively easy access to roads and numerous commercial centers, including Suva, the country's largest city. (Suva has a population of some ninety thousand, including perhaps ten thousand squatters.) Almost half of Fijians (45 percent as of 2005) live in urban or urbanizing communities. Under such circumstances, Fijians of all sorts are eating more nutritionally dense foods and are exercising less. Correspondingly, the health of Fijians is not good and is getting worse.

A comparison of BMI statistics collected in 1993 and 2004 appearing in the latest Fiji National Nutrition Survey indicated that "the proportions of overweight and obesity have worsened (increased) since 1993." Among people eighteen years of age and older, "overweight was 22% in 1993 and 32.3% in 2004; obesity was 9.8% in 1993 and 23.9% in 2004."[4] Moreover, among persons twenty and older, "borderline hypertension rates increased from 2.9% in 1993 to 7.2% in 2004, while hypertension increased from 9.8% in 1993 to 17.1% in 2004."[5] Although this report did not compare changes in the diabetes rates, another report issued in 2002 indicated that they were at 16 percent (11.5 percent of indigenous Fijians and 21 percent of Indo-Fijians), with the rates significantly higher in urban areas of the country (24.7 percent) as opposed to rural areas (12.8 percent).[6]

THE CASE FOR REGULATION: THE HOW AND WHY OF THE BAN

Although the health statistics do not seem to have improved since Fiji banned lamb and mutton flaps, most of the public health officials to whom we spoke (in New Zealand, Australia, and Fiji) thought the ban on flaps was an important step in the right direction. One particularly vocal supporter of the ban was Rod Jackson, the New Zealand-based epidemiologist who had been quoted in the *Independent* newspaper as saying that exporting flaps to the Pacific Islands was a form of "dietary genocide." When we interviewed Jackson in 2006 at his Auckland office, he emphasized that 75–85 percent of cardiovascular disease is caused by diet—by eating saturated fats and loading up on sugar-laden soft drinks. Though exercise may have health benefits, what is most important is what people put in their mouths.

From Jackson's perspective, the basic premise of public health is that water runs downhill. Therefore, if you want to change behavior, you have to make it easy for people to do so. For example, you have to find a way for people to feel satiated without consuming too many calories and too many saturated fats. Jackson hopes that genetically modified foods may eventually make this possible, but for now the easiest way to improve health is to channel consumer decisions in the right direction. Banning or heavily taxing foods with a high saturated fat content is a start. The taxes could then be used to subsidize the development of a local, healthy food industry. While New Zealand has moved to an open market, with tobacco and alcohol the only substances that are taxed heavily for health purposes, Jackson said that Fiji and other Pacific Island countries should do much more. Effective regulation is particularly feasible because the government of an island can readily monitor the products that are entering the country. He did not mention, however, that while small islands may be able to exercise physical control over their boundaries, they may not have much power internationally to challenge free-trade advocates like the WTO.

We began to understand some of the complexities in conversation with an indigenous Fijian veterinarian who was a member of the Agriculture Department at the time the ban was implemented. He explained that during the mid-1970s the meats allowed into Fiji (aside from beef and goat from Vanuatu) were from New Zealand and Australia. However, Fiji was getting primarily the cheap cuts that most people could afford, including lamb and mutton flaps. During the 1980s, as Fiji's chicken industry grew, there was a call to replace cheap meat from abroad with locally produced chicken. Yet the growing number of people living in towns continued to buy lamb and mutton flaps because they remained cheaper than Fijian chicken. During this time, health surveys began to indicate an increase in lifestyle diseases, particularly heart disease. Then, in the early 1990s, the ten-year quarantine that Fiji had placed upon a flock of imported Barbados Black Belly sheep was lifted. These were sheep adapted to the tropics that some in the Agriculture Department hoped would become the basis of an indigenous ruminant industry. Agriculture Department officials mentioned this finding to colleagues in the Health Department with the suggestion that a ban on the import of flaps might be a good idea.

All of these considerations persuaded Fiji's Minister for Commerce, Business Development, and Investment to take action. He implemented a ban, not on the import of lamb and mutton flaps, but on their sale in the country—a ban that would apply to all flaps, even domestically produced ones (which, according to Agriculture Department analyses, were actually leaner than those from New Zealand). He did so on the carefully worded grounds that flaps were "likely to cause the death of a person, or to injure, or to adversely affect the health or well being of a person."[7] As Fiji had acceded to the WTO's regulations in 1996, this phrasing, taken from Fiji's Fair Trading Decree, was designed to conform as much as possible to WTO specifications. Under the WTO category of "Technical Barriers to Trade," products can be regulated in order to protect human health and safety, as long as these regulations do not discriminate between trading partners or between locally produced and imported goods.[8]

Not surprisingly, these efforts to regulate or ban the sale of lamb and mutton flaps alarmed those with trade interests,[9] especially in New Zealand, the primary supplier of sheep meat to Fiji. Robert Hughes, a nutritionist who worked for the South Pacific Commission (SPC), told us that when he and his colleagues began in 1996 to study the role of fatty meat imports as contributors to the rising rates of obesity in Pacific Island countries, the New Zealand Trade Commissioner put direct pressure on the SPC to back off the issue.[10] Hughes also showed us a 1997 letter from the general manager of International Services of the New Zealand Meat Producers Board reminding him that "the Pacific region is an export market worth NZ$97 million FOB for New Zealand beef and lamb exporters. Consequently we would be most interested in learning more about the objectives and parameters of the Commission's study. We feel that establishing some dialogue on this matter could be mutually beneficial."[11]

Once the ban came into effect, and despite its careful wording, those with trade interests argued that there was no scientific evidence pointing to lamb and mutton flaps as inherently unhealthy. (It was not as if the meat came from animals infected by scrapie or other diseases.) They also argued that singling out lamb and mutton flaps as a health risk because of the high fat content was arbitrary, since many products, including butter and the corned beef produced in Fiji, contained as much if not more fat than flaps. All in all, they claimed that this ban "provided a really highly undesirable precedent in international trade" and should be challenged by the New Zealand government under the guidelines of the WTO.[12]

However, the Fijian government held firm, and the New Zealand government decided not to pursue the matter with the WTO. Part of the reason, according to an official we spoke with from New Zealand's Pacific Division of the Ministry of Foreign Affairs and Trade, was that Fiji presented New Zealand with concerns far more pressing than the ban. Ongoing ethnic conflict between indigenous Fijians and Indo-Fijians was challenging the country's fragile democracy. (Fiji experienced its fourth military coup shortly after we completed our 2006 research there.) In regard to the ban in particular, the official explained that, while the New Zealand government supported both free trade in general and the interests of the meat industry in particular, the trade in lamb and mutton was becoming an international liability. For instance, when Annette King, the former Minister for Health from New Zealand, had met with her Pacific Island counterparts, she frequently had encountered charges of hypocrisy. How could New Zealand be serious about promoting healthy lifestyles in the region when its export policy undermined the health of Pacific Islanders?

Moreover, the official explained, to the extent that the trade undermined the health of Pacific Islanders, it was becoming a domestic liability as well. It was widely known that New Zealand was providing medical services (including very expensive renal dialysis for diabetes) to patients from those Pacific countries with which New Zealand had both special relations and extensive trade (especially Tonga, Samoa, Tuvalu, and the Cook Islands). Indeed, such procedures were straining the medical budgets of urban hospitals in New Zealand. (It was reported, for instance, that it cost "about [NZ]$600,000 a year to treat overseas dialysis patients, mostly Pacific Islanders."[13]) One particular case had attracted intense controversy. Shortly before we began our study, the New Zealand press had given extensive coverage to a thirty-one-year-old

Tuvuluan man, married to a New Zealand citizen, who faced deportation because he had overstayed his visa. (There was also the added detail that he had assaulted and threatened to kill his wife.) Eventually the man was granted the right to remain in New Zealand because he had diabetes, and without the possibility of his receiving life-sustaining dialysis in Tuvalu, deportation, it was reluctantly concluded, would be a virtual death sentence.[14]

It may also be the case, we think, that New Zealand decided not to dwell on the ban because it did not have a large effect on New Zealand exports to Fiji. During 1999 (the year before the ban), the 10,200 metric tons of sheep meat exported to Fiji from New Zealand included only 211 tons of lamb and mutton flaps (in contrast, for example, to the 2,908 tons of forequarters, a less fatty, but still relatively inexpensive cut).[15] Indeed, New Zealand traders had told us that, though they were strongly opposed to the ban, lamb and mutton flaps had been only a relatively minor part of the sheep-meat trade into Fiji.[16]

The ban did go into effect relatively smoothly, with the Fijian government providing the public with advance notice and with information about the health risks of eating flaps. A graphic, thirty-seven-second television message produced by Fiji's National Centre for Health Promotion began in a forthright fashion with the narrator stating that when people bought flaps, they were buying fatty flesh—flesh, it was implied, that would become their own fatty flesh. Viewers were shown flaps, white with fat, placed in a pot of water on the stove. It was explained that when flaps were cooked and the water allowed to stand, the fat would float to the surface and harden. The water was then poured into a pitcher from which a woman's hand lifted out a great glob of congealed fat. Then, over successive diagrams of a healthy artery, a clogged artery, and a blocked artery, the narrator continued to explain that the fat would cause plaque to form inside blood vessels, making it harder for the heart to pump blood, and that when the artery closed up totally, a heart attack would be the likely result. The scene shifted to a middle-aged, stocky but not obese, indigenous Fijian man, probably a civil servant, climbing the stairs of an office building. Suddenly he bent over, clutching his chest. The narrator stated that if the

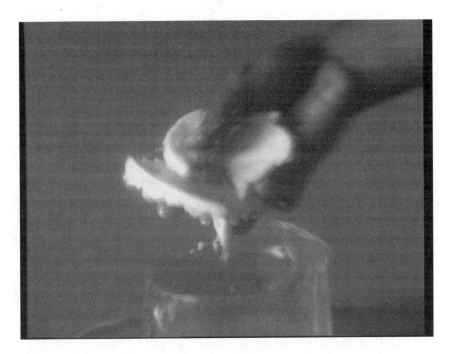

Figure 9. A scene from the Fijian television message concerning lamb and mutton flaps

clot broke and went to the brain, it could cause a stroke. Viewers then saw the man staggering as if he had just received a blow to the head. The final captions stated that "sale of lamb flaps will be banned in Fiji under the provisions of Fair Trading Decree, 1992" and exhorted viewers to "Cut down fat in your diet."

Such messages seem to have been effective in facilitating the ban. From what we could gather in conversation, and through 185 interviews we conducted in 2006 with the help of two social science graduate students from the University of the South Pacific, there was little public outcry. Few customers expressed confusion when they found that flaps were no longer available, and most Fijians accepted that the ban had been enacted for health reasons. The few letters-to-the-editor on this subject supported the prohibition as a health measure. One, in the *Fiji*

Times, was written by Susan Parkinson, a nutritionist and long-term resident of Fiji:

> I refer to your news item, "Ban on lamb flaps" (FT 11/12). From a health point of view, Cabinet has made a wise decision to prohibit the sale of this meat product in Fiji. Lamb and mutton flap is a by-product of sheep meat industries and is seldom sold for human consumption in developed countries. . . . Traditionally, many Pacific islanders enjoy the flavour of fatty meats and, for this reason, many purchase these meat products. The eating of fatty meats is one of the factors which leads to being overweight. The old saying "fat makes fat," is true when the extra calories provided by fat are not used up in exercise or keeping the body warm, as in cold climates. Because many modern people do not have the exercise needed to use up the calories from fat, they put on weight when they eat too much fatty meat, butter, margarine, and fried foods. Being overweight is a health problem because it often leads to the development of more serious illnesses in the form of high blood pressure, diabetes and heart disease—all of which are common in Fiji. Cabinet's decision to ban the importation of lamb flap will remove a low quality and unhealthful meat from the national diet.[17]

Parkinson and other Fiji-based nutritionists (as well as some of the people interviewed by the students) also told us that they hoped the ban would encourage the local production of more nutritious food. One assumption (which is shared by other analysts, including Rod Jackson in New Zealand) is that "traditional" foods are the most healthful and that if Fijians prefer imported foods, they are suffering from a postcolonial "inferiority complex," or they have been seduced by Western tastes. Nutritionists in Fiji note with concern that local fishermen come to the market in Suva, sell their fresh fish, and then buy canned fish to eat back home,[18] or that local people buy imported rice and instant noodles rather than indigenous taro.[19] Another dimension of the argument is that greater reliance on locally produced food promotes food security and economic development.[20] Hence the ban on lamb and mutton flaps fosters not only a more nutritious and secure diet, but also, for example, the development of an indigenous ruminant industry.

Yet, as desirable as a shift back to traditional, or at least locally produced, foods may be, the question immediately arises as to its practical-
ity. Fresh fish and taro cost more than canned fish and rice or noodles.
For cash-short Fijians, whether fishermen or urban dwellers, these less-
expensive choices make economic sense, at least in the short run. Moreover, despite the continuing effort in Fiji to advance the breeding of Barbados Black Belly sheep (now known as "Fiji Fantastic")—and the interest
expressed by a range of Pacific Island countries in acquiring stock—the
benefits are not likely to be seen for quite some time. When interviewed
in 2006, the veterinarian who played a major role in developing the animals estimated that, even under the best of circumstances, Fiji could not
hope to become self-sufficient in sheep meat for between twenty-five and
thirty years: "If you convert the amount of sheep meat consumed by Fijians into the number of animals you would need to supply that meat," he
said, "you are talking about incredible numbers." Such a commitment
would also involve diverting large amounts of land from other uses—a
point that has also been made in regard to expanding the local cattle industry. Finally, this veterinarian—and many others, nutritionists as well
as ordinary citizens—mentioned that, even with the ban in place, Fijians
seemed to be sicker than ever.

THE CASE FOR EDUCATION: FIJIANS AS CONSUMERS OF HEALTH

Of course, even with the ban on flaps, much land-mammal fat remains
cheaply available to Fijians. Another veterinarian, also a member of the
Department of Agriculture when the ban was put in place, told us that
he had been right to oppose it as ineffectual. Many poor people, he explained, just moved to the next cheapest sheep meat: to necks, shoulder-
chops, sausages, and the very fatty "curry pieces," not to mention tinned
meat.

The government of Fiji was well aware that more needed to be done.
In addition to the ban on flaps, it imposed a 10 percent tax on soft drinks,
and it has been educating people to make more healthful choices, as in

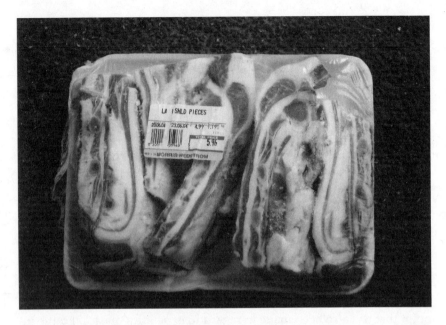

Figure 10.   Lamb shoulder pieces, often chopped into curry pieces, purchased in Fiji

the final message of the TV commercial to "Cut down fat in your diet." A similar effort to help people become informed in their choices was a poster distributed by the Ministry of Health entitled "What's in My Meal? Hidden Fat." The poster pictures plates of food commonly eaten in Fiji, including a pan-fried fish steak, a battered and deep-fried fish filet, taro with coconut cream, a chicken leg quarter with skin and without skin, a vegetable curry with rice, and a hamburger and fries. Under the plates are spoons, each representing 5 g of fat. Thus the chicken leg quarter with skin clearly has almost twice as much fat (20 g) as the one without skin, and the hamburger and fries have a great deal of fat (45 g) while the curry and rice have relatively little (10 g). The Ministry also placed health-focused messages in the phone book and on billboards in public places.

Such educational measures probably have had some beneficial effects. We did, for instance, see many overweight Fijians walking for exercise before and after work. And these measures may have prompted one

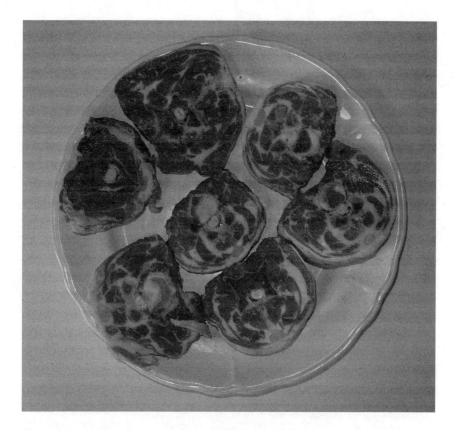

Figure 11.   Lamb neck pieces, purchased in Fiji

Pentecostal preacher in 2007 to challenge his indigenous Fijian parishio-
ners to control their weight. Expressing the rationale that your body is
God's temple, and God wants you to keep it healthy, he brought out a
scale and announced to his startled congregation (which included an
anthropological colleague) that he proposed to weigh everybody. He did
so, wrote down their weights, announced that some were definitely
obese, and urged those needing to lose weight to show progress at their
next weighing two weeks hence.[21]

These educational initiatives, whether in the form of exhortations from
the Ministry of Health or from the pulpit, did not present themselves as
repudiations of direct intervention or as alternatives to measures such as

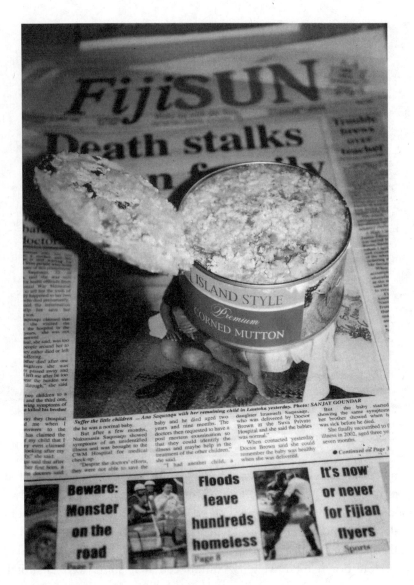

Figure 12. Corned mutton, canned and purchased in Fiji

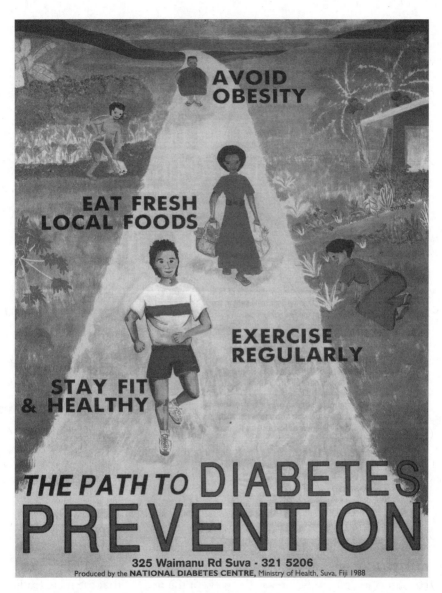

Figure 13. An insert found in Fiji's 2004 phone book (dated 1988)

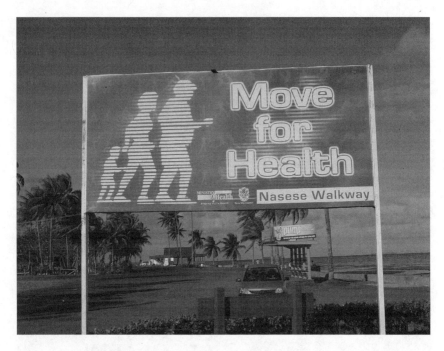

Figure 14.   A billboard along Suva's sea wall, where people are encouraged to take healthful walks

the ban on flaps or the tax on soft drinks. Instead, these spokespeople can perhaps be thought of as representing a middle ground, one that attempts to balance intervention with freedom of choice. Significantly, such a position could not be confused with a full-blown neoliberal agenda, according to which any decision, including one's choice of food, should be as private as one's choice of shoes. With its focus on the primacy of consumer choice, the neoliberal agenda is intimately linked to a view of the market as the most efficient mechanism to determine the availability and consumption of goods. This is the view of the market that the meat traders endorse: that meat never goes uneaten, nor should it. Aside perhaps from promoting educational initiatives that encourage more rational choices, governments should allow their citizens freedom of choice. But urging and assisting individuals, whether from billboards or the pulpit, to take greater responsibility for their health-related choices is a very different matter: it is an act of collective responsibility for a collective problem, not an effort to transform citizens into self-interested and autonomous consumers.

According the 185 interviews conducted for us,[22] most ordinary citizens do, in fact, seek a middle ground that balances intervention with free choice. Approval of the ban was not universal: 60 people opposed it, many of them claiming that it harmed poor people who needed a cheap source of meat. (Several suggested that if the government wished to prohibit anything, it might consider banning cigarettes.) And 22 expressed uncertainty, either offering no opinion or discussing both pros and cons. But 103 people said that the ban had been a good idea generally, because flaps are too fatty, and it is the government's job to protect citizens from products clearly deleterious to their health. Of these, 32 specifically mentioned, often emphatically, that they approved of the ban because it prevents inferior meat from being dumped on Fiji. Thus a twenty-five-year-old indigenous Fijian woman employed as an administrative assistant said that "flaps were too fatty and caused too many lifestyle diseases. Also, we must send the message to suppliers that we are not a dumping ground of their rejected meat." And a sixty-year-old Indo-Fijian man selling vegetables at a market said, "From my experience in New Zealand, flaps were only for dogs. They are a third-grade meat they're sending to us. They tend to dump these kinds of unwanted pieces on us."

Despite these differences, among all of the groups—those who supported the ban, opposed the ban, or were neutral—there were respondents (sixty-five in all) who specifically stated that people must also take responsibility for their own health choices. Thus one fifty-one-year-old indigenous Fijian woman who supported the ban said, "Yes, I support the ban because I heard in the media that this meat was bought from people who usually fed it to their dogs and was unhealthy. . . . [But] our health depends on us, on what we choose. I think the banning of flaps has made people become conscious of what is sold in the shops and what some foods can do to us, so that we can eat better, local foods." [23] Perhaps it is such a middle ground that needs more cultivation. Fiji's health statistics clearly have been getting worse. And while a majority of those interviewed said that the government should protect their health by whatever means necessary, few claimed that the ban on flaps had been successful in inducing Fijians to cut down on fat consumption. The ban has not solved the problem, and people are still making what would seem to be bad choices. If things do not change soon, most agreed, there will be many more sick Fijians straining the government's capacity to help take care of them.

FINDING WHAT WORKS

Jan Pryor, a physician and researcher at the Fiji School of Medicine, says that in Fiji and elsewhere in the Pacific there is a "clock ticking," and that a "fuse has been lit and a bomb is about to explode." With the "staggering numbers of NCD's [non-communicable diseases, another term for lifestyle diseases] striking younger and younger people within the country," the situation, he says, is dire.

Pryor is part of an international team engaged in a project to address these questions in Fiji and Tonga, and among Tongans living in New Zealand and Caucasians living in Australia. Focusing on adolescents (ages 13–18), Obesity Prevention in Communities (OPIC) is working to pinpoint the causes of youth obesity so that resources, which are always scarce, can be deployed effectively. Sponsored by a range of international organizations, OPIC is committed to finding out what works.[24] It seems to be striving for a balance between intervention and free choice.

We first learned of the project from Robert Scragg, the epidemiologist who was quoted in the newspaper as saying that "mutton flaps have caused more deaths in the Pacific than 30 years of nuclear tests" and who is OPIC's principal coordinator in New Zealand.[25] Scragg explained that OPIC grew from an earlier study of 3,275 New Zealand children (Pacific Islander, Maori, and "NZEO"—i.e., those of European, Asian, Indian, and other backgrounds). One of the findings of this study was that obesity is strongly correlated with skipping breakfast at home, presumably because hungry kids buy soft drinks and meat pies at the school canteen or from "tuck" shops.[26] However, further research was needed into the causes of obesity and how these causes might be addressed.

OPIC is designed to provide the needed research, largely through three kinds of "sub-studies." Economic sub-studies will measure the quality of life and model the costs of obesity (in terms of such variables as missed work and medical treatment). Such measurements and models can be important advocacy tools for health officials. Sociocultural sub-studies will involve in-depth interviews and questionnaires to explore patterns of eating, levels of physical activity, bodily self-image, and perceptions of others. These studies are intended to provide insight into how health might best be "marketed" in different contexts. Food policy sub-studies will determine how changes in food-related regulations (presumably including the Fijian ban on the sale of flaps and also the tax on soft drinks) will affect the supply of food and influence obesity. All of these sub-studies, according to Scragg, will "come up with the kinds of cost utilities—with the data and the arguments—that government economists demand concerning interventions into obesity."

We learned more about the OPIC project at a 2006 meeting of Fiji's National Health Promotion Council, at which two of Pryor's Fijian colleagues, both nutritionists, brought council members, including Fiji's two ministers of health, up to date on the project. First Jimaima Schultz provided background information. OPIC team members are working to determine the costs and benefits of various interventions, she said, and selecting effective interventions requires the right kind of information. The project team is investigating patterns of eating and exercise among Fijian youths, as well as the sorts of bodies these youths would like to have. The team is also investigating the extent to which commercial interests and advertising campaigns are contributing to overeating.

Gade Waqa followed with some of the specifics, largely about the sociocultural sub-study that has been completed and the interventions it has suggested. To begin with, she explained to the audience that they decided not to call the project Obesity Prevention in Communities, for fear of offending obese youth. Instead, they decided on Healthy Youth, Healthy Community. Concentrating on schools within the urban area of Nasino (near Suva), they sampled 1,500 Indo-Fijian and 1,500 indigenous

Fijian youth. At each school an "implementation committee" has devised a "plan of action" designed to reduce the frequency with which youth skip breakfast. They also promote eating fruit and other healthful snacks, encourage walking to school and other forms of exercise, and discourage watching TV and passive snacking on junk food.

The project team, Waqa continued, is also designing pamphlets to promote eating breakfast and has established a school-based breakfast program that features eggs (provided by the major Fijian egg producer). The team is also working with those in charge of school canteens to increase the healthfulness and reduce the costs of the foods offered there. It has arranged for media coverage on TV and in the *Fiji Times,* and for billboards encouraging people to choose healthy foods and to exercise regularly. The team plans to launch an intervention that encourages boarding-school students to plant their own vegetables. The students, Waqa emphasized, are already actively involved in creating their own strategies for making healthy choices. Concluding her presentation, she stressed that all of these efforts will be monitored by professionals to evaluate carefully the costs and to determine, through "a variety of exit measures," what the accomplishments have been relative to a control group.

In listening to these very competent presentations, we were aware, however, that there were likely to be departures from the plan. When we talked earlier with Jan Pryor, he expressed concern that his team was under great pressure to act rather than to investigate and deliberate. Given the ticking clock and the bomb set to explode, his team was forced to settle quickly on a set of specific interventions that could demonstrate a reduction in BMIs. The risk, of course, was that if data collection was inadequate, the interventions might be ineffective. For example, of all the measures they had planned, only the in-depth interviews had been completed.

For our part, we are not sure either about the OPIC interventions—but not only because the studies have not been completed. While entirely sympathetic to the commitment of the OPIC teams to deal with obesity in places like Fiji, we question if their epidemiological methodology is sufficient to address the complexity of the problem.

Our training as anthropologists makes us wary of interventions based primarily on the selection and correlation of restricted variables. Indeed, for variables to be counted and correlated with other variables, it is important to limit nuance and ambiguity.[27] For example, one measure that is significant to the OPIC researchers is that of skipping versus not skipping breakfast. In order for this to be a variable in Fiji's "obesogenic patterns,"[28] there must be clear indication of whether someone has skipped breakfast or not and whether that person has a BMI above a particular value. If these two can be correlated, then an effort is made to find a narrative that plausibly links the two. In this way, a statistical association can appear to be a causal link or explanation. Thus the link between skipping breakfast and obesity is provided by a narrative of students who satisfy their hunger by eating unhealthfully, either on their way to school or at school canteens. This narrative also suggests points of intervention, such as encouraging students to eat breakfast at home, providing breakfasts at school, or ensuring that school canteens offer more healthful foods.

We probed this breakfast-skipping narrative separately with Pryor and with Robert Scragg, both of whom told us that many studies have shown this correlation. However, while we were willing to accept for purposes of discussion that there is a relationship between eating breakfast at home and a moderate BMI, we wondered why this might be so. We wondered what eating at home means—whether in New Zealand, Fiji, or elsewhere. We became especially curious when we were told that the correlation held up regardless of what kind of at-home breakfast the children ate (e.g., whether chocolate sugar-bombs or oatmeal). Could it be that—depending on the place—eating breakfast at home fits into more complicated narratives that affect food consumption? And could these narratives be quite various? In a post-industrial society, for example, such a correlation might reflect class and occupational status. It might be, in such a context, that kids who eat at home in the mornings have at least one parent in attendance—one who does not have to go to work early. And eating breakfast might be correlated with more affluence, better-educated parents, and greater parental supervision.[29] But what of Fiji? We did not know, nor did Pryor and Scragg. Although they did not dismiss our general point, the fieldwork-based, qualitatively oriented methodology necessary both to generate and probe such alternative possibilities was clearly not part of their approach. It would not only complicate understandings, but perhaps hold up interventions. And yet the interventions themselves seemed to depend on what appeared to us as restricted variables placed within seemingly straightforward narratives.

But let us accept for the moment the narrative that the OPIC team uses to link skipping breakfast and obesity. This narrative, as we have mentioned, suggests several interventions, some of which seem easier to enact than others. Improving canteen food or providing breakfasts at school would not be difficult; the principal challenge would be to make healthful food choices appealing and affordable (following Rod Jackson's public health model of water flowing downhill). Encouraging students to eat breakfast at home seems to be a more difficult proposition. The OPIC study did seek in its in-depth interviews to determine the variables accounting for skipped breakfasts. The second draft of the "Report on Interviews with Indigenous Fijian and IndoFijian Youth" says that of the 48 indigenous Fijians and 48 Indo-Fijians interviewed, "many . . . skipped breakfast, especially Indo-Fijian girls. The most common reasons given . . . were 1) insufficient time, and 2) not feeling like eating. Most participants who said that they were rushed in the mornings either got up late and/or had to leave home early." One Indo-Fijian male reported, "I wake up late or rush to school. Interviewer: And why do you wake up late? Participant: Because I sleep late (laughs). Interviewer: So that's the basic reason why you skip breakfast? Participant: Yes. And also I don't feel like eating in the morning. Interviewer: So you tend to cover it up during the day or at recess or lunch? Eat much more? Participant: Yes." [30]

The project team concluded that children who skip breakfast also lack time and appetite in the morning. But why? If the team wishes to plan an effective intervention that will encourage kids to eat breakfast at home, the reasons that they do not might usefully be probed further. And this would be hard to do without a more in-depth study. Was this Indo-Fijian boy up late at night studying? Was he, for instance, under pressure by his parents to do well in school and thereby get a good job upon graduation, either in Fiji or abroad (perhaps in New Zealand)? And was he snacking to stay awake while he studied and therefore not hungry when he woke up? And might the girls skip breakfast for reasons that are different from those of the boys?

Certainly, according to the report, skipping breakfast seems far more common among Fijian girls than boys, and gender is much more reliably correlated with breakfast practices than ethnicity (i.e., indigenous Fijian or Indo-Fijian).[31] Perhaps some insight into the life circumstances of indigenous Fijian girls can be gained from the work of the anthropologist and psychiatrist Anne Becker about the relationship among body, personhood, and society in the Fijian village of Nahigatoka. During 1988, Becker began long-term research which taught her (among other things) that large bodies were, in "traditional" Fijian culture, aesthetically appealing. Such bodies indicated that a person had a capacity for hard work and also that a person was fed and cared for by a large social network: "The display of core cultural values through the medium of personal bodies is a primary expression of the ethos of care within the social body. The body is the showplace of its caretaking community. Social relationships in Fiji are fundamentally mediated through the exchange and distribution of food. Care, or *vikawaitaki*, is manifested in food exchange and feeding, and subsequently in bodily form. . . . *Vikawaitaki* is the quintessence of virtue and marks the body with the record of its success."[32]

At least in the 1980s, few girls were anxious about their weight, and most ate a great deal. However, Becker's subsequent work in 1998 in the town of Nadroga showed that the situation had changed. In an approach that fruitfully combined the qualitative methods of an anthropologist with the quantitative ones of an epidemiologist, Becker traced the effects on indigenous Fijian girls of "the sudden infusion of Western cultural images and values."[33] She argued that three years after the introduction of television, these girls had come to see a slim figure as necessary to success in the modern world. Moreover, they had come to believe that they were personally responsible for reshaping their bodies—for losing weight. Of the thirty girls in Becker's sample, 74 percent reported feeling too big and fat, and a significant number of "those who watched TV at least three nights a week were 50% more likely to see themselves as too fat and 30% more likely to diet."[34]

Yet these girls still found themselves in contexts of heavy eating (and of calorie-dense foods, including fatty meats, that are more and more available in modernizing Fiji). They were still encouraged to eat a great deal by elder kin whom they would offend if they did not partake, for example, of the foods prepared for the usual family Sunday dinner. They were caught up in an impossible situation: they became dissatisfied with their bodies; they felt like failures because they remained fat (often with BMIs above 35); they could not diet systematically for fear of alienating kin and abrogating core cultural values of community care; and they—some 15 percent—began to engage in extremely unhealthful patterns of disordered eating, such as binging and purging.[35]

We suggest that comparable factors, grounded in the complexities of modernizing sociocultural life among indigenous Fijian girls, were responsible for some of the skipped breakfasts in the OPIC study.[36] Although it is unlikely that Becker's analysis of such factors would apply equally well to all of the adolescents studied by the OPIC team, we think that her kind of context-rich interpretation would usefully augment and inform the epidemiological studies of OPIC.

That being said, we are also aware that the predilection of anthropologists for such studies makes it far easier for them to critique a plan of action than to devise one. Although we are skeptical of the narrative in which eating breakfast at home has been placed, we respect the commitments of those trying to find out what works. And if interventions such as convincing parents to insist that their children eat breakfast at home, offering breakfast in school, and providing healthier canteen food actually do address the ticking time bomb of Fiji's diet-related health problems, we will happily congratulate the OPIC team.

THE BAN THOUGHT THROUGH CRITICALLY

Most of those promoting health in Fiji, including members of the OPIC team, stressed that individuals must learn to take responsibility for their own health, both for the sake of their ultimate well-being and to help alleviate the burdens on the national health care system. The "Health

Promotion Policy for Fiji" proposed by the National Health Promotion Council (and submitted as a bill for government approval shortly after our 2006 research) stated that its primary objective was to enable "people to increase control over and improve their own health."[37] While emphasizing personal responsibility and choice, the policy also recognizes that at least limited governmental regulation is necessary because "some people are able to . . . [make such healthy choices] and others [particularly children] are not."[38] Consequently, the policy proposes "that the Ministry of Education implement the School Nutrition Policy and require head teachers and school principals to limit the availability of junk food sold to children on school premises."[39] But concerning the food more generally available to adults, the policy is modest. It proposes only that nutritionally informed labeling be required, although only on prepackaged foods (whether locally produced or imported). Concerning such labeling, it calls for conformity with the various international standards, including the requirement that there be "statements on the various type of fat content."[40] Such labels would give the fat content of meat, such as canned corned beef or canned mutton, that enters the store already packaged, but no information would be provided about meat, such as lamb curry pieces or necks, that is wrapped at the store. To judge from documents of this sort and from our conversation with public health professionals, this is about as far as the Fijian government is likely to go. The government's ban on the sale of lamb and mutton flaps seems to have been a one-off event. Certainly, a government committed, as the Asian Development Bank describes it, to policies aimed at "boosting private sector development . . . through structural reforms to promote investment and the private sector" is unlikely to flout the WTO and international lending agencies with additional trade bans.[41] It is, to be sure, difficult to predict the actions of the present coup-based and confrontational military government, which came to power in 2006. However, the declines in Fiji's textile industry (because of Asian competition), the problems in the sugar industry (because of an aging infrastructure and the likely withdrawal of an E.U. subsidy), and the setbacks in the tourist industry (because of the coup) may make the country sensitive to the possibility of international economic sanctions.

Nonetheless, the ban on lamb and mutton flaps was, we think, an important event—one that remains worth thinking about by a variety of differently located Fijians and Pacific Islanders more broadly. While the ban did little to affect the high rates of lifestyle diseases or to stimulate local production, either of traditional foods or of import substitutes, it seems to have been effective in other ways. Whether by design or accident, the ban was strategic in doing both a little and quite a bit.

The ban did little to inconvenience many Fijians. Lamb and mutton flaps were only a minor part of their diet, and inexpensive cuts of meat are still readily available. At the same time, the ban did quite a bit to demonstrate that the government had the power and the will to act in the interests of its citizens. (As such, perhaps the ban also projects the unity of an ethnically divided nation as well as the unity of the nation with the state.) Moreover, the ban did quite a bit to urge Fijians to be mindful of what they eat and, more generally, to be mindful of what is "good enough" for them and their fellow countrymen. Significantly, by asserting that flaps were not good to eat, the ban did quite a bit to project Fiji's international position. As part of the critical scrutiny that flaps compel, the ban made a strong and reverberating statement in a regional dialogue. Fiji was not to be dumped on by powerful neighbors. It would stand up to New Zealand and Australia and would not allow its people to eat what these regional First World powers feed to their dogs. In so doing, Fiji also established itself as unlike Papua New Guinea, whose government did not have the will or the power to reject such inferior items and whose people both craved and needed them. It presented itself as a model for other Pacific Island nations, such as Tonga, that are looking for solutions to their pressing problems.

TONGAN TRADITIONS

The only Tongans with whom we spoke about the traffic in fatty meat were attending a 2004 meeting in Auckland of the Heart Foundation of New Zealand. The occasion was to announce the findings of a study concerning the consumption of a fatty, brined beef brisket—*povi* or *pulu masima*—primarily by Samoans and Tongans living in New Zealand.[42] The Heart Foundation had wanted to explore health issues among Pacific Islanders living in New Zealand. That the study ended up concentrating on *povi/pulu masima* was, however, the decision of Pacific Islanders themselves.

At the meeting, some thirty-five Pacific Islanders—nutritionists, dieticians, educators, pastors, and community members—gathered to learn the results of the study. Mafi Funaki-Tahifote, the Tongan dietician in charge, began by outlining the history of *povi/pulu masima*—a history echoing the one we had heard from meat traders. Salted beef was first brought to the Pacific by explorers, whalers, and missionaries and quickly became a high-ranking food—and one with significant ceremonial value—because imported foods were more prestigious than indigenous ones. Brined brisket is still given by individuals and families to fulfill obligations and show respect, and this beef is still one of the mainstays (ranked second only to pork) of church and family feasts in Samoa and Tonga. It is a highly valued food in celebrations that strengthen the bonds of kinship, express community solidarity, and help maintain the cultural traditions and social ties that constitute identity. Yet, Funaki-Tahifote continued, *povi/pulu masima* may well be a contributing factor (along with consumption of other fatty meats and lack of physical activity) to the serious health problems of obesity, diabetes, and cardiovascular disease that Pacific Islanders face both in New Zealand and at home.

In the discussion that followed Funaki-Tahifote's presentation, a number of issues recurred. Central among these was the degree to which people can change their traditions—especially ones so obviously important (indeed definitional) as the giving, receiving, and consuming of ceremonially appropriate food. Several participants stressed that culture is not static; culture is what we make of it and should not be used as an excuse to avoid responsibility for changing our behaviors. Another countered and proposed what proved to be the dominant view of the participants: that *povi/pulu masima* is part of their roots. Although communication and education can increase awareness of the health hazards, there is no alternative. It is inexpensive and delicious and an important part of who they are. The best they can do is to cook it differently so as to eliminate some of the fat.[43]

Throughout the discussion as well as in the subsequently published report,[44] there was agreement that the diets of Tongans and Samoans had shifted so that meat protein was no longer merely a supplement to a meal of carbohydrates and vegetables but had become the central component. Indeed, the written report described Tongans and Samoans (especially those living in New Zealand) as binging on protein—especially, given economic constraints, on cheap protein. Along with brined brisket, the cheap proteins of significance that were frequently mentioned in both the discussion and the report were Kentucky Fried Chicken and lamb and mutton flaps.

Of this fatty trinity, lamb and mutton flaps seem the most compromised: only flaps were described as dumped. Only flaps were described (as by the Prime Minister of Tonga) as "hardly edible." In fact, lamb and mutton flaps are generally singled out in arguments that the Tongan government should regulate imports so as to address Tonga's truly appalling rates of lifestyle diseases. Thus, as part of a recommendation that the Tongan government place a quota on the import of all fatty meats—eventually to reach 50 percent of the 2002 import volume—two government consultants, Boyd Swinburn and Mark Lawrence, referred to lamb and mutton flaps in particular:

> For mutton flaps alone—2002 imports into Tonga were approximately 3 million kg. which is approximately 500 g per capita per week. Mutton flaps contain approximately 40 g fat/100 g, half of which is saturated fat, and 420 kcal. Reducing the consumption of mutton flaps and other fatty meats by 50% and replacing it with the same amount of fish (about 3 g fat, mostly unsaturated fat, and 120 kcal per 100 g) would therefore reduce fat intake by over 30 g/day, saturated fat by over 15 g/day, and energy intake by over 200 kcal/day. . . . The health gains . . . would result from reducing the consumption of fatty meats (due to a 50% reduction in supply). Further health gains and reductions in NCDs [noncommunicable diseases] would come from other components of the National Plan to reduce NCDs such as programs aimed at increasing physical activity and reducing meal sizes.[45]

This recommendation of a quota on fatty meat imports, especially on lamb and mutton flaps, was designed not only to confront Tonga's health issues, but also to conform to Tonga's position in a broader political economy. Tonga was hoping to join the WTO but needed the sponsorship of New Zealand and Australia (the major exporters of lamb and mutton flaps) to do so. Tonga's strategy was that of its closely watched neighbor, Fiji. It sought to restrict trade in ways that conform to WTO regulations: to provide documentable health reasons and to avoid discriminating against any particular exporting country. However, despite the proposal's careful wording, the recommendation of a quota was tabled by the Tongan government, lest it compromise the support of New Zealand and Australia for WTO accession.

The recommendation was also shaped by the realities of what has been called a MIRAB-based political economy (Migration, Remittances, Aid, and Bureaucracy)—one that Tonga shares with some other Pacific Island countries (though not with Papua New Guinea or Fiji). As the anthropologist Mike Evans makes clear,

> Large-scale migration of islanders from the South Pacific to a variety of locations (most notably Australia, New Zealand, and parts of the western United States) has resulted in significant flows of cash and material from overseas migrants to kinspeople remaining in their natal areas (that is, *Mi*gration and *R*emittances). Foreign-aid donations have also resulted in the movement of large amounts of resources into South Pacific states and underwritten the development of sizable government bureaucracies (that is, *A*id and *B*ureaucracy). Taken together the flow of resources through these two main channels has had profound effects on a number of South Pacific microstates.[46]

In effect, Tonga runs on remittances and on aid.[47] Because economic activity focuses on aid-dependent bureaucracies, urban centers are flourishing at the expense of the increasingly underpopulated countryside. This means that the traditional agricultural resource base is underutilized, and there is increasing dependence on imported food. In this situation, lamb and mutton flaps as cheap protein cannot easily be subjected to a total ban. Because flaps are likely to remain an important source of food in Tonga, the best that can be hoped for is regulation through a quota.

In fact, nothing to date has come of the recommendation to place a quota on flaps, and experts on the country seem to think that, with WTO accession, Tonga will have even less regulatory latitude. Be that as it may, it is the case (as we saw in Fiji) that Tongans eat many fatty things. Why all the focus on flaps?

It is true that flaps constitute the single largest household expenditure in Tonga for purchased foods (followed by chicken pieces, white bread, and corned beef).[48] And it is true that flaps are eaten far more frequently than is *pulu masima*—which is almost twice as expensive and is eaten most often at feasts.[49] But we believe they are singled out not just because they are imported and consumed in such large amounts. After all, flaps were singled out in Fiji even though they were imported and consumed in relatively small amounts.

As we have suggested, flaps occupy an interestingly ambiguous place in what might be called a system of fatty foods. They are located between the cheap fatty meats that constitute world-traversing, highly caloric, branded and patented fast foods and the cheap fatty meats that constitute regionally distinct, highly caloric, ethnic foods. They are unlike, say, KFC chicken, which is popular among both white people and Pacific Islanders and is never described as being "dumped" on Tongans.[50] Lamb and mutton flaps are also unlike brined brisket, which is also never described as being "dumped" on Tongans.[51] Although white people do not eat it, Pacific Islanders have inscribed *povi/pulu masima* with significant and distinctive sociocultural meanings. This leaves lamb and mutton flaps. Because white people do not eat them, and Pacific Islanders (with the possible exception of Papua New Guineans) do not imbue them with great sociocultural meaning, flaps become the repository not only of health concerns but also of postcolonial anxieties.

In thinking about the special salience of flaps, it is instructive to note a somewhat comparable import. Turkey tails, most of which come from the United States, flood many parts of the Pacific, including Tonga (though not Papua New Guinea or Fiji, where tariffs protect local poultry industries).[52] Although turkey tails have serious health implications and are not eaten by those who export them, they do not seem to be fetishized as flaps are. In our view, flaps draw most of the heat because they are associated with the more proximate First World powers of New Zealand and Australia.[53] They are more readily seen as both the product and the symbol of seemingly inextricable relationships of dependency— relationships that are at the heart of the heat.

CONCLUSION One Supersize Does Not Fit All

FLAP VERSUS MAC

The controversy about lamb and mutton flaps is not likely to go away soon. In fact, things were heating up again in 2007. Pete Hodgson, then the New Zealand Minister of Health, was under pressure from his Pacific Island counterparts (as were his predecessors) to do something rapidly to help Pacific Island peoples lead healthier lives. Perhaps, some Pacific Island health officials suggested, New Zealand itself might limit the export of fatty meats, especially lamb and mutton flaps. To respond appropriately to such pressure, Hodgson's ministry, together with the Ministry of Foreign Affairs and Trade and NZAID (New Zealand's agency of international aid and development), commissioned a report about the "impact of the New Zealand export of sheep meat (mutton and lamb) flaps on obesity and chronic disease in Pacific Island countries."[1] Issued in March 2007, much of this report remains confidential (with all of its recommendations redacted). It did, however, provide some interesting data: 29 percent of New Zealand's lamb and mutton flap exports during 2006 went to the Pacific Islands;[2] the trade was worth between NZ$24 and $28 million in 2005; and the quantity of flaps exported to Tonga had doubled between 1976 and 2005. In addition, the report acknowledged "that there is not a significant market for sheep meat flaps in their countries of origin."[3]

In August, 2007, the Health Committee of New Zealand's Parliament released another report, entitled "Inquiry into Obesity and Type 2 Diabetes in New Zealand." Although the report concentrated on the health of people living in New Zealand, it did consider ways to improve the health of people living in the Pacific Islands. The majority of committee members recommended "that the Government, the New Zealand Meat Industry, and the Pacific nations work cooperatively to phase out the export of fatty meats (such as mutton flaps), to Pacific nations."[4] A minority disagreed with this recommendation, however. While granting that obesity and type 2 diabetes contribute significantly to rising health care costs, this minority insisted that these problems had to be addressed on the level of individual motivation and choice: "The emphasis should be on practical approaches that change attitudes to food and exercise.[5] The necessary changes in diet and exercise habits will not occur through Government pressure."[6]

In its formal response to the Health Committee report, the government rejected the majority recommendation to phase out the export of flaps.[7] While not disputing that flaps were harmful when eaten too frequently, it argued that consumers would only replace flaps with another fatty meat product. It also claimed "that an export ban could also raise questions, whether from other countries or domestic interests, regarding New Zealand's international obligations."[8] In other words, such a ban would compromise New Zealand's commitment to free trade. Members of the meat industry applauded the government's position. One spokesperson had expressed fears to us that the industry would end up as a scapegoat again: "It would be crazy and naive to blame the whole Pacific obesity problem on just one food."

It is indeed true, as we have seen in Fiji, that banning flaps may not improve the health of consumers, perhaps in part because they can just switch to another fatty meat. The fact remains, however, that flaps are not just another fatty meat; they have a salience—both material and symbolic—that curry pieces, canned corned beef, and even turkey tails (not to mention KFC's pieces and McDonald's burgers) do not. As fatty flesh that some relish and others feed to their dogs (and to which few outside of Papua New Guinea have been able to add much value), flaps invite a critical scrutiny. They encourage many Pacific Islanders to think critically about the broader relationships that distinguish the eschewers from the eaters, the First World from the Third, the white from the brown. Because flaps reveal such relationships within a global life process, they resist commercial efforts to resubmerge them into the anonymity of circulating commodities, subject to the supply and demand of consumer choice—to make them just another meat that someone will eat when the price is right. Because no one grows a sheep for its flaps, flaps make a lot happen. Flaps may be exported, but they just do not go away.

ON MAKING GOOD CHOICES IN TONGA

As we have seen, many advocates of free trade, including those in the meat industry (both in New Zealand and Australia) believe that the Pacific Island preoccupation with flaps is unfortunate and misplaced. Consumers, they argue—whether in New Zealand and Australia or in Papua New Guinea, Fiji, and Tonga—should be allowed to choose what they want and can afford, and the issue gets blown out of proportion by people who choose to eat too much of what would otherwise be a good enough food. From their perspective, the global omnivore's dilemma of what to eat should be solved with a little common sense.

Some tales from Tonga seem to support this perspective. International press reports about the recent death of the king of Tonga in 2006 emphasized not only his gigantic size, but also his sensible decision to mend his ways. Here is one account from the *Washington Post*: "At age 14, the future king was one of Tonga's top athletes; he played tennis, cricket, rugby, and also rowed competitively. In the 1990s, Tupou IV led his

108,000 people on a diet and exercise regime aimed at cutting fat in a nation where coconut flesh and mutton flaps are dietary staples.[9] From a weight the *Guinness Book of Records* listed as heaviest for any monarch, 462 pounds, the king shed around 154 pounds."[10] Comparably, recall our story about the affluent, 290-pound Tongan woman who ate least 2 kg of lamb and mutton flaps (an extraordinary 8,400 calories per day in flaps alone, by our calculation, assuming the flaps were boneless, with about 40 percent of these calories coming from saturated fats).[11] This woman confronted the problem and reformed her eating habits after her doctor predicted an early death. "Instead of letting a maid do the cooking," she said in her interview with the Japanese journalist, she took charge of her meals to "completely change [her] diet."[12] For breakfast, she ate only one papaya, one slice of toast without butter, and a cup of lemon grass tea; for lunch and dinner she ate a small amount of fish, salad, and fruit.

Both of these tales of unrestrained excess—especially on the part of the socially privileged—encourage readers to shake their heads in wonderment.[13] Surely no reasonable person would eat quantities even remotely that large. After all, flaps are not like tobacco and heroin, which are addictive and harmful in any quantities. What took the king and the woman so long to come to their (common) senses? In tales of this sort, the problem is not with the lamb and mutton flaps but with those who choose to eat them—and lots more—to excess. Perhaps some people might benefit from additional education and encouragement, but, unless they are incapable of making mature choices, change is essentially a matter of their personal choice.

In the *Washington Post* article about the king, we learn that he was not only attempting to rectify matters for himself (though apparently too little, too late, as he died soon after, likely from complications linked to obesity) but also encouraging other Tongans to follow his lead.[14] The 290-pound woman was also trying to take responsibility, although the article did not indicate if her efforts to lose weight were successful.[15] It did say, however, that other Tongans were having considerable difficulty with self-regulation and reported the discouraging results of several weight-loss competitions that Tonga organized for its citizens. The first, in which 983 people participated, ran from August 1995, to January 1996.

Once registered, [the] weight, height, and other physical conditions [of the participants] were checked. After that, their weight was checked every month and they individually received instructions on their diet and exercise. They were told to exercise [at least] 30 minutes a day, try to reduce sipi [lamb and mutton flaps] and increase fish in their diet, to eat more vegetables and fruits instead of sweets. . . . Out of all the people registered for the 1st competition, . . . 661 resigned half-way without losing any weight. In any country, it is surely difficult to change [the] usual diet to go on a healthy one and to keep regular exercise.[16]

Difficult as such self-reform may be, the moral of such tales is that it is up to those who eat themselves into such messes to diet themselves out of them. Just do it!

Even those free-traders who understand that it may be difficult to "just do it" are likely to reject any policies that they see as infringing on individual choice. This was the case for those members of the Health Committee who wrote the minority opinion mentioned above. Their view was that of the New Zealand National Party, which "stands for freedom, choice, independence and ambition, . . . [and believes in] less government not more red tape, . . . [and is] against political correctness and strongly for personal freedom and responsibility."[17] Rejecting the recommendation that the export of lamb and mutton flaps to the Pacific Islands be phased out, they advocated instead "an approach that identifies and successfully targets the socio-cultural aspects of the problem. In western, Maori, Pacific Island and Asian cultures, food is often central to social interaction, and a mark of hospitality. Basic attitudes to food have to change before the tide of overweight and obesity begin to reverse. Our 'cultural hard drive' has to alter, so that healthy choices are the choices of preference. . . . National is not in favour of food and drink policies . . . that remove individual choice."[18]

We find this perspective instructive in the degree to which it is massively equalizing: all people are alike in their capacity to choose and to struggle to make hard choices that may go against cultural norms. There may be special cases—particular configurations of the "cultural hard drive"—but there are no exempting cases. This position is presented as principled. Perhaps in the manner of the aphorism commonly associated with Voltaire's philosophy of freedom ("I disapprove of what you say, but I will defend to the death your right to say it"),[19] the position defends the right of all not only to make good choices, but also to make bad choices—including the choice to eat the flaps that the more enlightened would never choose for themselves. The position is also presented as practical. If, for instance, Tongan cultural standards concerning food-centered interactions contribute to obesity, it is up to Tongans to figure out how best to shift their basic attitudes.[20] After all—at least according to the information widely disseminated when the king of Tonga died—he took personal responsibility. Through exercising will power and dieting, he, and his subjects, could learn to approximate the good health of their (collective) youth. This was true regardless of how and whether flaps came to their shores.

However, in our view the issue is whether a focus on the importance of choice should prevent us from examining the contexts in which choices are made. It may be the case that the king of Tonga was able to stop making bad choices (just as he would have been able to pay for dialysis if necessary). But does this mean that ordinary Tongan citizens have the same range of opportunities?[21] Moreover, should a focus on the importance of choice preclude a channeling or curtailing of the choices available? Perhaps, indeed, the Tongans should not be told what to eat. But does this mean that the government of this MIRAB-dependent people should not be allowed the choice to restrict certain imports—regardless of their contribution to New Zealand's economy?

THE POLITICS OF PERSONAL CONSUMPTION

Such a choice-focused politics is, of course, promulgated widely in the United States. Consider, for example, the Web-based activities of the Center for Consumer Freedom (CCF), a nonprofit organization dedicated to promoting personal responsibility and protecting consumer rights. The CCF is funded by various food companies and individual consumers committed to defending the "right of adults and parents to choose what they eat, drink, and how they enjoy themselves."[22] To this end, the CCF, among other campaigns, advocates against warning labels on food and lawsuits that target companies whose products are believed to cause obesity. Their literature and press releases rail against the "growing cabal of 'food cops,' health care enforcers, militant activists, meddling bureaucrats, and violent radicals who think they know 'what's best for you' [and] are pushing against our basic freedoms."[23] Vigilant in the defense of these rights, the CCF scans the media to reveal or discredit the actions of this growing cabal. Among its most effective—and engaging—Web-postings are cartoons, including the one shown in figure 15, reprinted from the *New Yorker*.[24]

What makes this cartoon funny is the degree to which it demonizes perfectly ordinary ingredients that so many enjoy. From the perspective of the CCF, the teacher in the cartoon is a food cop—albeit disguised as caring and good-natured—indoctrinating children about monstrous pepperoni! Those who categorically oppose regulation might continue by noting that if this teacher's school served pizza at all, it might well require official approval. Such, at least, was the case in Texas, where in 2005 the legislature was forced to abridge school nutrition policy with what came to be known as the "cupcake amendment," which allowed cake and pizza to be served on special occasions (e.g., a child's birthday).[25] Most of the CCF's cartoons, we think, present attempts at food regulation as so extreme as to be ridiculous. And the next step from the ridiculous is the malign.

In this regard, we were alerted by the CCF through an e-mail message on January 4, 2008, about ominous "breaking news." One of four articles cited was "Europeans Chafe Under New Year 'Nanny State' Laws," reporting that "Europe [that is, Germany, France, and Portugal] started 2008 with a raft of new laws against smoking, air pollution and even junk food adverts, but some grumbled that the New Year's resolutions from the 'nanny state' cramped their style." These laws, justified in terms of "public health costs," were leading to "an ever more coercive control over our private lives."[26] Thus efforts at regulation are either caricatured as ludicrous by the CCF or portrayed as potentially grave curtailments of personal freedom and responsibility.[27]

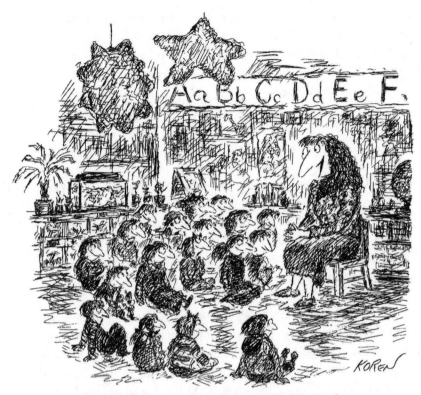

"Once upon a time, there was a frozen pizza, and inside the pizza some very bad monsters lived. Their names were refined white flour, reconstituted tomato, and processed cheese. But the worst monster of all was called pepperoni!"

Figure 15. Cartoon from the *New Yorker*, reprinted with permission of Cartoonbank.com

The CCF may go further in its use of ridicule—and perhaps in its definition of what constitutes a fundamental threat to freedom—than many opponents to food regulation. However, those about whom we are aware (largely) agree that eating and good nutrition should remain a private matter and that the exercise of personal responsibility is within the capacities of most people. Simply by following common sense, people will make reasonable choices: what is out there to buy is healthful, if eaten in moderation. Because pizza and cupcakes, soft drinks, and McDonald's meals are acceptable when consumed in moderation, regulations such as elimination of soda machines in schools, reduction of the trans-fat and caloric content of school lunches, and the expansion of nutritional labeling are, according to this logic, not only unnecessary but also infringements of basic freedoms.[28]

COMMON SENSE CONSUMPTION?

Such arguments taken at face value—as apparent common sense—serve to sustain the status quo as an unexamined given. This certainly is the view of many influential food writers and activists who consider the status quo—business as usual—to be unsatisfactory. At the least, they argue, if people are to be expected to make reasonable choices, they must be informed concerning what these choices entail.

Thus, Eric Schlosser in *Fast Food Nation* and Michael Pollan in *The Omnivore's Dilemma* (previously mentioned) agree that there is much about the contemporary food system (which brings us pizza, cupcakes, soft drinks, and McDonald's meals) that needs to be illuminated and challenged—that needs to be defetishized.[29] Schlosser discusses the environmental effects of industrial agriculture, the labor conditions under which products such as hamburger are processed, the substances added to enhance taste and appearance as well as increase shelf life, and the consequences to health of frequent and long-term consumption. And Pollan demonstrates that much of our diet, including the syrup to sweeten our soft drinks and the feed to fatten our hamburger-destined cows, depends on the excessive use of fertilizers and pesticides. Both Schlosser and Pollan want to provide consumers with the knowledge necessary to exercise appropriate caution and restraint—to make reasonable food choices that further personal and planetary health.

Independent filmmaker Morgan Spurlock also wishes to defetishize our contemporary food system. He does so, less through argument than through dramatic demonstration of the effects of living exclusively on McDonald's meals for thirty days. In his Academy Award–nominated film *Super Size Me,* he recorded his metamorphosis from a healthy man into a one-man public health crisis.[30] He limited himself to McDonald's food and the Coca-Cola beverages it served; he ate three full McDonald's meals every day; he chose every food offered on the McDonald's menu at least once during the 30-day period; he picked a McDonald's salad once in ten meals; he opted for the "super size" portion (substantially larger quantities available for a minimal extra cost) whenever it was offered; and he tried to walk no more than 5,000 steps every day—as (apparently) the average American does. On this regimen Spurlock took in about 5,000 calories daily, about 3,000 calories more than the average requirement of a man his size and with this activity level. By his estimate, in 30 days he ate roughly the same amount of McDonald's food that the typical American would eat in 8 years. During the course of the month, Spurlock gained 24.5 pounds and increased his BMI from a "normal" 23.2% to an "overweight" 27%. He also experienced mood swings, heart palpitations, and sexual dysfunction, and he sustained irreversible liver damage. The doctors who monitored him expressed surprise at his rapid deterioration. In effect, through a sort of fast forwarding, Spurlock became the "everyman" in the worldwide community of fast-food consumers, the iconic (or totemic) product of the nasty little secrets hidden within our ordinary, taken-for-granted, industrially produced foods.

Spurlock's experiment, targeted as it was at McDonald's, drew the company's immediate response that his food choices had been atypical and unreasonable in their complete lack of moderation. However, one of Spurlock's points was that McDonald's, with its supersized offerings, hardly encouraged moderation. It should be mentioned that, after the screening of Spurlock's film in 2004, the company did withdraw supersized fries and beverages from its restaurants—but only to introduce in 2006 Coca-Cola's 42-ounce, 410-calorie soft drink, the "Hugo."[31]

Indeed, moderation in consumption would hardly appear to be the objective of fast-food and soft drink companies. In this regard, McDonald's ambition to sell as much as possible—an ambition reflected in its aggressive marketing and its supersized options—would seem to be matched by that of its collaborator, the Coca-Cola company. In his examination of the Coca-Cola company, anthropologist Robert Foster quotes a 1996 address to shareholders in which the Chairman and CEO of Coca-Cola (from 1981 to 1997) explicitly set out the goal of making its product preferable to water: "We have become increasingly mindful of one undeniable fact," he said, that "the average human body requires at least 64 ounces of liquid every day just to survive, and our beverages account for not even 2 of those ounces. For every person on this planet consuming at least 64 ounces is not an option; but choosing where those ounces come from is."[32] His conclusion: that Coca Cola was "resolutely focused on going after the other 62." Foster comments wryly, "the global expansion of soft drink consumption is a war against tap water or, more accurately, the transformation of tap water from an end product to an ingredient."[33] (It might be noted that the forty-two ounces in Coke's Hugo are just twenty-two ounces short of the per-person target.)

Schlosser, Pollan, and Spurlock do important work in describing how our food system operates. They demonstrate that, under contemporary conditions in which companies work hard to sell us foods that may be unhealthful to both people and the planet, it is difficult but important for consumers to exercise informed choice and moderation. They also raise issues of public policy that should be addressed. For instance, Schlosser shows that worker safety at American meat-processing plants needs to be ensured through more consistent enforcement of state and federal labor laws; Pollan shows that the farm subsidies on which the corn-based American agro-industrial complex depends need to be reevaluated; Spurlock shows that schoolchildren need to be protected from too easy availability of fast foods. However, all of these arguments largely challenge the status quo in its own terms: people, if properly informed, will choose as consumers to say "no" to products that jeopardize their health and their environment; people, if properly informed, will choose as citizens to say "yes" to policies that provide for the safety of workers, the effective use of public money, and the health of children.

Thus, these food writers tend to engage in a politics that emphasizes personal choice. Despite different motivations and objectives, they are speaking much the same language as opponents of serious food regulation such as the National Party and the Government of New Zealand and the CCF in the United States.[34] In perhaps the most synoptic statement of this politics, Pollan concludes his latest book, *In Defense of Food,* with this advice to the discriminating omnivore: eat no food your grandmother would not recognize as such, eat in moderation, eat mostly vegetables.[35] But, we ask, how far can you go with the politics of personal choice? The likes of farmers' markets may be great places for some to find recognizable food, but can such markets feed the differently positioned people located across the globe? Can, more specifically, such a politics of personal choice effectively address the omnivore's dilemma in the Pacific Islands?

ON STIGMATIZED FOODS

As we have shown throughout this book, for many in the First World, lamb and mutton flaps are a stigmatized food. Some will, of course, spend their Saturday afternoons turning them into barbecued specialties. Others will, without doubt, order them at one of the few upscale restaurants that serve fatty meats as transgressive novelties. Nonetheless, most white people will not eat them with any regularity because they are too fatty. When we have shown pictures of flaps—both raw and cooked—to friends and students, most respond with disgust. Not so to Big Macs—regardless of class distinction and despite Spurlock's efforts. Although it may be the case that the human body cannot tell the difference between one kind of fatty meat and another (and Big Macs do have lots of fat—about 29 g in the five hundred or so calories in each one), they remain different both perceptually and politically. A consumer in what we have called a "flap food nation" bears a very different totemic identity from one in a fast-food nation. Consequently, the king of Tonga and Spurlock are supersized evocations—everymen—of rather differently positioned groups.

Thus the Tongan prime minister could plausibly (if controversially) refer to flaps as "hardly edible." To do so would be to defend the inherent worth of significant numbers of his people. However, the president of the United States could not plausibly refer to Big Macs in the same way. To do so would be to diminish the inherent worth of significant numbers of Americans. The former statement would be regarded as concerned and populist; the latter, as snobby and classist. In other words, while flaps might readily (though, again, controversially) be described as dumped on Pacific Islanders, Big Macs would never readily be described as dumped on Americans.[36] (Imagine the response, for example, if we recommended that Americans and others in the First World stop eating Big Macs and feed them to their dogs instead, or if we were to purchase a Big Mac in public and feed it to our dog.) In these regards, fast foods (despite the efforts of Schlosser, Pollan, and Spurlock) just sink back into the pool of commodities that—with help of advertising and branding—jostle with each other for consumer dollars. For example, as a recent British article attests, "Evidence shows that fast-food restaurants are thriving despite campaigns to promote healthy eating. McDonald's is selling more burgers than at any time since it arrived in Britain 34 years ago. . . . There were over 88m visits to McDonald's restaurants around the UK last month [December 2007] alone. The figure is up by almost 10m on the previous year, or an average of about 320,000 more each day. Sales are growing at close to the fastest rate since the late 1980's."[37] We do not know precisely how to account for the growth in McDonald's sales in the United Kingdom (or elsewhere, as sales have been going up all over the world), and we imagine that there are various sociocultural reasons, depending on where the restaurants are located.[38] However, we imagine the appeal is similar to that of flaps: of repletion through the eating of an inexpensive and fatty meat in a convenient, modernist setting. There are, of course, those who wish to prevent the proliferation of fast-food restaurants in Britain (especially near schools) and throughout the world. However, the fact that McDonald's burgers, and hamburgers in general, are eaten by members of most ethnic groups, most races, and (no doubt, with different frequencies) by most socioeconomic classes means that they themselves are seen as politically neutral, if not necessarily good for you. This is to say, to be a member of a fast-food nation is too universalistic to be a totemic identity. McDonald's burgers are, generally speaking, taken for granted and, if left to themselves, many people will continue to eat lots of them. Moreover, those who strongly criticize them may appear as borderline killjoys. Therefore, the only regulation we can imagine (and advocate) would be to limit child-focused advertising and school-focused availability.

Flaps, of course, are not ubiquitous, and therefore they stand out as marking difference. They remain compellingly totemic and capable of provoking ongoing critical thought about First World and Third World relationships and global life processes. Flaps, as we have said, are not only trouble, but troubling. As such, they will not shut up. This is the case, most generally, because the totemic identity that flaps compel is thoroughly ambivalent: that of a second-rate modernity, one constituted by second-rate food that can make people sick. And many Papua New Guineans, Fijians, and Tongans are made uncomfortable by this identity: they smile and shrug, they try a ban, and they fail to implement their regulatory plan.

AND SO?

To be sure, flaps will get eaten when the price is right. Yet the ambivalences and complications of their sale into the Pacific Islands make the trade far from just a matter of supply and demand in a global economy. There are claims and counterclaims concerning the free trade in flaps. Who (if anyone) is dumping, and if so, on whom? And more broadly, who owes what (if anything) to whom?

As anthropologists, we believe it is our job to contextualize all of these claims and counterclaims. Most generally, we have shown why human beings are attracted not only to meat but also to fatty meat. And we have shown why fatty meat, at least for those not sufficiently affluent and well-educated to temper their desires, may be associated with the good life—with celebration and repletion. More specifically, we have explored as thickly as possible the implications of the commercial reality that sheep are never grown for their flaps, but that the flaps are commoditized nonetheless. We have conveyed how flaps become an entrepreneurial opportunity for traders who develop, nurture, and cope with their often difficult Pacific Island markets. We have conveyed how variously positioned Pacific Island countries respond to their circumstances as "flap food nations." We have conveyed how the health of Pacific Islanders may be affected by the trade, both the undernourished Joseph and his son in Papua New Guinea and Tupou IV's overnourished subjects in Tonga. We have conveyed how health professionals (epidemiologists, physicians, and health educators) ponder and struggle with the problems they attribute to the consumption of flaps. And we have conveyed how the politics of personal consumption may not be effective enough to influence the structures that bring flaps (and the like) to some and not others. This is to say, we have described what flaps make happen, including a critical scrutiny of the relationship between those who eschew, eat, or ban them.

Throughout, it has been our hope that all of those caught up in this tangle of talk and activity will think, if they read this book, that we have given them a fair hearing, although not necessarily an uncritical one. If so, then they may become convinced that we are giving others a fair hearing also. They may then be inclined (whether farmers, meat processors, meat traders, government officials, epidemiologists, or the range of flap consumers with whom we have worked) to listen to others and perhaps to accept that the others deserve consideration—to grant that others should be taken seriously. This is to say, we have tried to remain responsible to our various and often multisited constituencies. Yet, as we argued at the beginning of this book, in addressing issues of public significance—after moving between all of our various constituencies—we must also accept our obligation to struggle toward a position that conveys a policy.

We do appreciate the difficulties faced by New Zealand as well as Australia with their relatively small, export-focused economies. While the policies and practices of free trade they embrace are not ones we would necessarily regard as ideal, they are pursued, as far as we can tell, with commendable transparency and consistency. Correspondingly, we do not fault those in the meat industry in New Zealand or Australia—and certainly not the meat traders—for trying to sell what they produce. The meat industry is highly competitive, and all parts of the animals must be sold to make a profit. We do not think it is reasonable to expect the New Zealand government to restrict the export of flaps to any particular place.

We also should say that the appeal of cheap meat, including fatty meat, is undeniable to many in the Third World. Nutritionally dense and often hard to come by, it not only tastes good but also has the allure of modernity. When available at affordable prices, it will be consumed with gusto.

That flaps are nutritionally dense may, of course, both enhance and diminish the health of those who eat them. Based on our Papua New Guinea research, we think that overall, and at least under present circumstances, the trade in flaps is beneficial for many undernourished and protein-deprived people. For Joseph and his family, a feast of flaps was a special luxury, and one we were happy to contribute to. Finally, in defense of the trade into Papua New Guinea, we note that locals are increasingly offsetting the stigma of flaps by incorporating them into multiple dimensions of their lives.

That flaps are nutritionally dense does, however, contribute to the problems other Pacific Islanders may be having with obesity and attendant health issues. This is not to deny that these health issues have many causes. Certainly they are not the result of one product alone. To place such blame runs the risk of being arbitrary and ineffectual. In this regard, the ban on flaps in Fiji seems to have selectively (though minimally) disadvantaged some commercial interests while doing little directly to bring the country's obesity problem under control. However, we do think that this ban did have some useful results. Among the positive aspects of Fiji's self-assertion as a flap-free zone was that it suggested to Fijians that their government was (at least at this time) concerned about their welfare and that their nation was capable of asserting its sovereignty against substantial external pressure. In addition, the ban (like the exhortations of the Pentecostal preacher) was a dramatic reminder to Fijians to exercise more care in what they eat. Finally, the ban may have facilitated other potentially valuable interventions, such as those promulgated by the OPIC team. Although as anthropologists we found the explanatory narratives generating these interventions to be rather thin if not unconvincing, and we would seek to know much more about the Fijian contexts affecting whether schoolchildren do or do not eat breakfast at home, we would be delighted if the interventions do work—for whatever reason.

Tonga—the country we know least well—faces extraordinary difficulties. With their MIRAB economy and their dire health conditions, Tongans are flummoxed by flaps—and by other cheap, modernist foods. Given these circumstances, we think that considerable latitude should be given to Tonga for regulatory experimentation. We recognize that most New Zealanders and Australians in the meat industry—including those trading into the Pacific Islands who were especially generous in helping us with the project—would disagree strongly. As we have granted, it may be unreasonable to expect New Zealand to ban exports of flaps to the Pacific Islands. But this does not mean that it is reasonable for New Zealand to insist on blocking Tonga's attempts, as part of a multifocal approach, to regulate fatty meat imports.

Certainly it must be acknowledged that many Tongans are far less well placed in the free market than most meat processors and traders (many of whom are, as we have seen, the success stories of the free market). For this reason alone, Tonga should be free to try whatever it can— whether quota or ban (whether consistently or inconsistently applied to all fatty foods)—to deal with a set of interrelated, life-threatening, and intractable problems. Some, like the CCF, would argue that if people do not take personal responsibility, they deserve what health problems befall them. However, our position follows the previously mentioned perspective of the epidemiologist Rod Jackson: for there to be any real change in Tongan eating habits, good food choices must be made as easy as possible. This is the case even if this means regulation by a "nanny state." After all, Tongans are already regulated by their MIRAB dependencies. These are, we think, the dependencies—and attendant vulnerabilities— that lead Tongans (and other Pacific Islanders) to speak about the dumping of lamb and mutton flaps—to speak about being dumped on by those who should do better.

And so, we call for some forbearance and recognition of claims based on a moral, not just a market, economy. We who are relatively advantaged should make our politics an acceptance of theirs, allowing Pacific

Islanders (Tongans, Fijians, Papua New Guineans, and others)—whose thinking about flaps has contributed to their critical understanding of the world—to exercise the choice of leaving the Pacific Island family of "flap food nations." They ask all of us to weigh in with our support for them—not to push them too hard.

Notes

1. We should also mention that there are now large markets for flaps in China, Mexico, and Africa. Flaps are sold into Europe, often to be used in "donner kebabs." Our focus is on the Pacific Island trade, which is far more controversial, partly because of the serious, diet-linked health problems there.

2. Although there is a technical distinction between lamb and mutton, the terms *lamb flaps* and *mutton flaps* are often used interchangeably among the public, and so we use the combined term to encompass the range of usages.

3. For tomatoes, see Brandt 2002; green beans, Freidberg 2004; broccoli, Fischer and Benson 2006; papayas, Cook 2004; pineapples, Richter 1985; and coffee, West, n.d.

4. For chickens, see Dixon 2002, and Striffler 2005; on chickens, pigs and cows, Stull and Broadway 2004; fruit, Martin 1990.

5. See, especially, Llambi 1993; McMichael 1994; Kneen 1999; McKenna, Roche, and Le Heron 1999; and Bonanno 2004.

6. A peripheral but thought-provoking version of this story, about an exquisite morsel for the wealthy and refined, is provided by Theodore Bestor (2001; 2004), who has mapped the migration of Atlantic bluefin tuna as they are rushed from run-down ports in New England to elegant sushi restaurants in Japan.

7. Pollan 2006.

8. Thus, according to a recent syndicated article in our local newspaper, Twinkies,™ the "beloved little snack," contain thiamine mononitrate made from Chinese petroleum. According to this article, eight of the ingredients in Twinkies come from domestic corn and three from soybeans. But "there are others—including thiamine mononitrate—that come from petroleum, Chinese petroleum. Chinese refineries and Chinese factories." This revelation was especially disquieting, given that toxic adulterants from Chinese factories had just been discovered in pet food and toothpaste (Ettlinger 2007, A6).

9. Sullivan et al. 2003.

10. In fact, the Anglican Bishop of the Solomon Islands, Terry Brown, reports that such noodles "represent one of the most widespread changes in SI [Solomon Island] diet over the last twenty years—one barely sees kumara [sweet potato], yam or taro sup-sup [soup] any more. Obviously this contributes to some health problems" (e-mail communication, June 6, 2007). Anthropologist Karen Brison finds that "Maggi noodles are the new staple food at least among the Fijian families I have stayed with" (e-mail communication, June 6, 2007). For an analysis of the attraction of instant noodles among Fijians, see Vatucawaqa 2002.

11. This information is from a recent survey by *Forbes* magazine; see Altucher 2007. In these countries, between 78.4 and 94.5 percent of adults above the age of fifteen are considered overweight by the World Health Organization. *Overweight,* as measured by the World Health Organization, means having a body mass index (BMI)—a ratio of height to weight—equal to or greater than 25. *Obesity* means having a BMI equal to or greater than 30. There are several problems with this measure. An important one is that large-boned people, other things being equal, are heavier than small-boned ones. A more accurate measure of those at risk for the development of lifestyle diseases is adiposity—a ratio of fat to body mass. But this measure requires more precise and therefore expensive appraisals.

12. Again, we are focusing only on those flaps that go to the Pacific Islands, not elsewhere.

13. We received this e-mail on April 1, 2008. In addition to his academic credentials, Dr. Walter Willett is also the author of *Eat, Drink and Be Healthy* (2001).

14. Health officials in Pacific Island countries may, of course, be engaged with the international scientific literature about the potential health risks of certain additives.

15. See Gewertz and Errington 1991.

16. Richter 1985.

17. See Errington and Gewertz 2004.

18. Clifford Geertz explains the distinction between a thin description and a thick description with references to winks, twitches, and parodies of winks and twitches. A thin description equates them all as simply rapid contractions of the eyelid. A thick description contextualizes each as having a different significance in social life (1973, 3–30).

19. For elaboration of the difficulties of multisited research, see Hannerz 1992; Marcus 1995; and Foster 2002.

20. See Gewertz and Errington 1991 and 1999; and Errington and Gewertz 1987.

21. These were or had been students at Papua New Guinea's Divine Word University, who were also employed at Nancy Sullivan, Ltd. to work as anthropological consultants.

22. We took careful notes throughout our interviews, and the quotations we provide are as accurate as we could make them in the absence of a tape-recorded record.

23. We should mention that all of those with whom we dealt on this project are, relatively speaking, benign; they are not, for instance, those who traffic in arms, body parts, or adulterated drugs.

CHAPTER ONE

1. Differently located people compare the foods on their plates to those on others' plates—and, in so doing, create politically salient distinctions. Certainly such was the case among the plurality of Jewish sectarians that Feeley-Harnick describes, who, during the intertestamental period, distinguished themselves from each other as appropriately godly through their various foodways: Essenes from Sadducees, from Christians, and from others. Who ate what, where, when, how, and with whom—all defined these groups relative to one another. Although Feeley-Harnik asserts that "gastronomy is geography" because "foods are intimately linked to the place-times of their growing, making, and eating" (1981, xvi), she also makes clear that such gastronomies and geographies are never static because, as comparative, they are always political. Foods travel, people travel, and food systems shift. As

they do, they carry with them what has become an increasingly global politics.

2. For the "man the hunter" argument see, especially, Lee and Devore 1968. For its "woman the gatherer" corrective, see Dahlberg 1981.

3. Hart and Sussman (2005) convincingly demonstrate the problems with such a stereotype and argue that early humans were more often hunted than hunters.

4. This is not to deny that our ancestors were undoubtedly eaten by other predators; see Rose 2001. Hart and Sussman (2005) elaborate this point; they also argue that our ancestors were more hunted than hunters to the extent of significantly downplaying the importance of meat eating in human evolution. They are virtually alone, however, in making this argument.

5. In fact, contemporary chimpanzees hunt meat with apparent enthusiasm, and meat, in some contexts, provides 20–30 percent of their caloric needs. See Stanford 2001. Dominguez-Rodrigo (1997) suggests that our early ancestors may have acquired a considerable amount of meat through active scavenging, either by chasing carnivores away from their kills or by finding carcasses that had died from natural causes. This is to say, they did not rely exclusively on gaining meat from abandoned and well-picked-over carnivore kills.

6. Wrangham et al. (1999) provide this early date.

7. Even if cooking entered the scene more recently, its initial effects would still have been significant. See Leonard 2002.

8. Wrangham et al. 1999.

9. Leonard 2002.

10. Smil 2002, 204; see also Aiello and Wheeler 1995.

11. Leonard 2002, 67. For comparable arguments, see Foley and Lee 1991; Foley 2001.

12. Eaton, Eaton, and Konner (1997), suggest that for Paleolithic humans, protein intake was typically above 30 percent in daily energy.

13. Speth and Tchernov 2001.

14. Leonard 2002.

15. Smil 2002.

16. These kills might include those of the relatively recent late Pleistocene (of 20–10,000 years ago), when horses were driven off cliffs.

17. Speth and Spielmann 1983.

18. Smil 2002, 606.

19. Smil 2002, 606–7. Larsen also discusses this transition under the heading "The Agricultural Revolution: Less Meat, More Plants, Less Nutritional Density" (2003, 3894S).

20. Some of these same social connections and cosmological associations may be made through the exchange of plant foods, such as vegetables. However,

even these vegetable exchanges may often be linked with meat exchanges. Thus, among the Wamira of Papua New Guinea, men are made anxious by their dependence on women's fertility and sexuality and seek to redress the balance through the ritualized exchange of surrogate children in the form of both taro and pigs. One without the other will not do. See Kahn 1986.

21. Schieffelin 1976.

22. As Conklin makes clear in her ethnography of mortuary cannibalism among the Wari (2001), when deceased relatives offer themselves up for consumption in the form of white-lipped peccaries, they do so partly in reciprocity, in gratitude to their living kin for having shielded them from the abandonment of death by ritually ingesting their (often decaying) human bodies.

23. Genesis 1:26.

24. Fiddes 1991, 2.

25. Vialles (1994) illustrates this transformation from animal to edible in her excellent structuralist analysis of French slaughterhouses. For more on the ways in which animals are categorized, see Leach 1972; Fiddes 1991.

26. Engels, quoted in Fiddes 1991, 165. This point is consistent with Mintz (1985), who argues that, during the early Industrial Revolution in Britain, most of the animal protein available to working-class households went to the primary worker, generally the senior male. The other members of the household survived on sugar and flour—usually as treacle and bread.

27. Smil's figures for Britain and France are of carcass weight without specification of species. Consequently, as he fully recognizes, these figures do not directly indicate how much meat people actually ate, even on average. The amount of edible meat varies according to species—chickens and pigs produce a higher proportion of (potentially) edible meat than do cows. And carcass weight does not itself indicate the extent to which the carcass was actually utilized—the extent to which, for example, edible offals were likely consumed. In order to estimate how much meat was actually consumed in Britain and France, we have reduced the carcass weight by one-third, assuming that in Europe a mix of species was eaten and as much of the carcass as possible was consumed. This extrapolation allows approximate comparison to the figures Smil provides for the United States, which are of trimmed weight (though exclusive of the offals, which would push the figures for actual consumption somewhat higher). This extrapolation also allows comparison with the (approximated) figures for the preindustrial periods.

28. Horowitz 2005, 22.

29. Sobal 1999, 187.

30. These statistics are summarized in Smil 2002, 612–613. Again, we have transformed carcass weight into edible weight by reducing the figures by one-third.

31. Drewnowski 1999.

32. Mahler 1995.

33. Horowitz 2005, 17 and 130.

34. Note, however, that the "game our ancestors ate was much leaner than today's domesticated meat: a venison steak derives 82 percent of its calories from protein and 18 percent from fat, whereas a choice sirloin cut derives 84 percent of its calories from fat and only 16 percent from protein—proportions that are virtually reversed" (Eaton and Shostak 1986, 9).

35. Harris 1985, 41. See also Speth and Spielmann 1983.

36. The appeal of fatty meat when cooked may be further enhanced as the meat is browned—caramelized—as through roasting or frying. Pleasing aromas and flavors are released through the Maillard Reaction, which involves the recombination of the protein molecules denatured by heat and sugar molecules released from the meat by heat.

37. Some claim that as many as 90 percent of our taste buds respond to fat. See Fletcher 2005; Laugerette et al. 2005; and Abumrad 2005 for discussions of a fat taste receptor in rodents. See also Herness and Gilbertson 1999 and Petersen 2005 for data about fat taste receptors in humans.

38. This analysis follows from Harris 1985.

39. McGee 2004, 131.

40. Horowitz 2005, 22.

41. Horowitz 2005, 86. Although these recipes also called for adding as much water as possible, the sausages were no doubt vastly superior to those made from rotted and verminous meat famously described at the same time by Upton Sinclair in *The Jungle* (2001).

42. Such definitions of what constitutes appropriate levels of fat are, as we will explore, subject to numerous influences, including those from various sectors of the meat industry. Thus, as one example of an effort to increase the marketability of meat laced with fat, during the U.S. agricultural recession of the 1920s cattlemen sought to enhance the desirability of the heavily marbled meat from corn-fed, purebred beef. Central to this effort was Alvin Saunders, editor of the *Breeder's Gazette,* whose strategic work culminated in the U.S. Department of Agriculture initiating a grading program in 1927 based on visible marbling. The USDA criteria—criteria still in place—gave top rating to the most heavily marbled: designating it as U.S. Prime. For more, see McGee 2004, 136. Also, see Ufkes for a discussion of how the development of a leaner pig was "propelled by changes in consumer demand and crisis and competition in U.S. meatpacking" (1998, 251).

43. Indeed, some have argued that, even under circumstances of ample nutrition, fat may not produce satiation. For example, Blundell and MacDiarmid

suggest that foods "high in dietary fat have a weak effect on satiation, which leads to a form of passive overconsumption, and a disproportionately weak effect on satiety (joule-for-joule compared with protein and carbohydrate). This overconsumption . . . is dependent upon both the high energy density and the potent sensory qualities (high palatability) of high-fat foods. A positive fat balance does not appear to generate a tendency for behavioral compensation, and there appears to be almost no autoregulatory link between fat oxidation [fat metabolism] and fat intake" (1997, 63). However, Heatherington and Rolls, while citing some evidence in support of the idea that "fat may be less satiating calorie-for-calorie than carbohydrates," conclude that "this proposition is yet to be examined systematically" (1996, 284).

44. The argument is that eating fatty meat produces "a pleasure response modified by what scientists call 'the endogenous opiod peptide system'" (Sims 1998: 11).

45. Mintz 1985, 208.

46. Holland 2005.

47. See "Barbecue Lamb Belly the Slow Way," n.d. One irony of doing research in a global world where people garner information from each other's Web sites is that such data about New Guinea come from a post stimulated by our own Web inquiries concerning lamb flaps. See Rex 2005.

48. Bruni 2007.

49. The literature on lifestyle-related diseases in the Pacific is extensive. The comprehensive volumes by Jansen, Parkinson, and Robertson (1990) and by Coyne (2000) are especially informative. See also Temu 1991; Hodge, Dowse, and Zimmet 1996; Simmons and Mesui 1999; Lako and Nguyen 2001; Taufa and Benjamin 2001; Temu and Saweri 2001; Gill et al. 2002, Evans et al. 2001 and 2003; Hughes 2001 and 2003; Hone and Haszler 2004; Curtis 2004; and Hughes and Lawrence 2005.

50. Swinburn 2004.

51. According to the "thrifty gene" hypothesis, certain ethnic groups, Polynesians included, possess genes that evolved to maximize metabolic efficiency under conditions of food scarcity—as during long sea voyages. These genes predispose members of these groups to lifestyle diseases when conditions of food scarcity are lifted and they can eat all they want. For a general elaboration, see Neel 1962, and for a Pacific Island application, see Pryor 1976. The thrifty gene hypothesis is by no means accepted by all researchers. Many social scientists see it as grossly reductionist, arguing that "the cognitive, emotional, and psychoneuroimmunological effects of colonialism and genocide that link indigenous peoples worldwide" play more important roles in the development of diabetes than any genetic basis (Ferreira and Lang 2006, 17). On the other hand, many medical

researchers see it as too simplistic from a genetic perspective to account for the variable susceptibility of different populations to lifestyle diseases. These researchers think that genes play an important but exceedingly complex role. For one example of the complex role genes play in the occurrence of diabetes in different populations, see Diabetes Genetics Initiative of the Broad Institute of Harvard and MIT, Lund University, and Novartis Institutes for BioMedical Research 2007. As one expert in the subject of "nutrigenomics" at the University of Michigan explained to us, fetuses become adapted over long periods of time to the diets of their mothers. This may adversely affect the functioning of their insulin-producing beta cells when, as adults, they are confronted with new kinds of foods under conditions of modernity (Burant, e-mail communication, February 5, 2008).

52. The article, written by Atsuko Yamamoto, appeared in *UNO! Magazine* during the late 1990s. It was translated from the Japanese and sent to Robert Hughes, a nutritionist working for the South Pacific Commission. He gave us a copy when we interviewed him in Brisbane during 2006. We have no independent verification that the woman described was, in fact, eating what was reported, although we have no doubt that she was eating a lot.

53. South Pacific Consumer Protection Programme 1997.

54. Concerning differences in kind: it is not just that Donald Trump has quantitatively more money than most other Americans; rather, he has a qualitatively different range of choices—including how to respond to serious illness—and set of life possibilities.

55. See in particular Karl Marx's "labor theory of value" (1906).

56. See especially Baudrillard 1981.

57. Daniel Miller (1988) calls this "consumption work." See, also Callon, Meadel, and Rabehariosa 2002, for a discussion of the way commodities are "qualified" and "requalified" as they move along commodity chains. For a sophisticated summary and application of such perspectives, particularly as they apply to such branded products as Coca-Cola, see Foster 2008.

58. Foster calls such a process "critical fetishism": "a heightened [and analytic] appreciation for the active materiality of things in motion" (2006, 285). Although Foster appropriately promotes this perspective for academic analysts, we see local people engaged in it as well. See, for an elaboration, Gewertz and Errington 2007.

CHAPTER TWO

1. See Calder and Tyson 1999, 165.

2. Established in the early 1920s, the Meat Board had, by the 1970s, grown into an extremely powerful organization. This power is illustrated by an account

of a famous conversation offered by one participant's son: "Sir John Ormond (Chairman of the Meat Board) and my father (Sir Jack Acland, Chairman of the Wool Board) were brothers-in-law. Uncle John was very charismatic, very definite, very thump the bloody table. Dad was much quieter, so they were an excellent combination. And when they really wanted something from government, they went up together. Once they went to see Henry Lang, who was Secretary of Treasury, and [Finance Minister] Muldoon was there. He was very rude and abrupt and John Ormond said, 'Sit down, Muldoon, sit down. You do not control this country, Jack Acland and I control this country.' " (Acland, quoted in Calder and Tyson 1999, 11).

3. The creation of new, domestically owned processing plants was restricted. Thus, while the long-established, British-owned plants were allowed to continue to operate, the giant U.S. processors were blocked from entry. The subsidies and price supports included subsidized credit; grants to encourage pasture development and its stocking; subsidies for fertilizer, weed control, and irrigation structures; and generous "supplemental minimum payments" on the sale of each animal. These payments reached a peak in 1984 at 67 percent of the price farmers got for the sale of their lambs. For more about these subsidies and price supports, see Calder and Tyson 1999, 105–8, and Harris and Rae 2006.

4. Maugham summarizes the long-term instability of this position: "The only way the system could be kept going was by making large compensatory payments to the farming and export sectors, by extensive overseas borrowing, and by more and more regulation" (1998, 30).

5. Another problem from the perspective of the meat processors involved labor. They felt squeezed by unionized slaughtermen and other workers at plants whose (already high) wages escalated and whose industrial actions routinely occurred at the busiest time of the slaughtering season.

6. These reforms also inaugurated a process that eventually reduced the power of labor unions in meat plants and elsewhere. Workers lost much of the power of collective action and many of the protections of arbitration. By 1991, with the passage of the Employment Contracts Act, all prior union-negotiated awards and agreements were declared invalid, and the relationship between employees and employers was defined as no different from any other commercial contract.

7. Aerial fertilizing—top-dressing—of pasture had been subsidized by the government, and the subsidies often were greater than the costs of the work, so that farmers sometimes actually made money directly from the government subsidies.

8. In 2004, the Organization for Economic Cooperation and Development estimated that the incomes of sheep growers were subsidized by only 3 percent in Australia and 1 percent in New Zealand (Australian Bureau of Agricultural

Resources and Economics and the New Zealand Ministry of Agriculture and Forestry 2006, 42).

9. In New Zealand and Australia there was a period of transition in which both whole and disarticulated carcasses were on the market. Hence, at the time of Finlayson's spectacular deal with the Soviets, there were both undesirable carcasses and undesirable cuts for which markets had to be found.

10. On agriculture in Australia, especially as it has been transformed by neoliberal reforms, see Lawrence 1987; Lawrence and Vanclay 1994; Lawrence 1999; Harris 2003; Anderson 2004; Pritchard and McManus 2000; and Pritchard 2005a and 2005b. For a comparison with New Zealand, see Burch et al. 1999 and Harris and Rae 2006.

11. Barrett 1987, cited in Stull and Broadway 2004, 69.

12. See Horowitz 1997.

13. Stull and Broadway 2004, 65–81.

14. Industry Commission 1994, 175, 175, 199, and appendix H, 120.

15. Calder and Tyson 1999, 288.

16. In 2000, the Employment Contracts Act was replaced by the somewhat more labor-friendly Employment Relations Act. Nonetheless, the power of the unions remains significantly diminished.

17. Aotearoa is the Maori name for New Zealand.

18. Calder and Tyson 1999, 288.

19. For additional information, see Emergency Response and Research Institute 1991.

20. See Wratten 2002.

21. See Bird and Norris 2006.

22. At the time of this research, NZ$1.00 was worth about US$62.

23. Hayman 2006, n.p.

24. For more about the problems of forging such multicultural communities, see Errington and Gewertz 2004, 109–37.

25. Brian Hayes, in his remarkably informative and witty book, *Infrastructure*, writes that "trying to get into a meat-packing plant is like trying to penetrate the CIA" (2005, 106). It is, thus, to the credit of Donald Stull and Michael Broadway that they were able to make repeat visits to at least one of the plants they describe in *Slaughterhouse Blues* (2004).

26. Halal slaughtering demands that sheep be alive when their throats are cut. New Zealand animal-protection laws demand that the sheep be unconscious prior to slaughter. Hence, electrical shock is calibrated to stun but not to kill. Indeed, tests are run periodically to insure that the stunned animal is able to regain consciousness. We might mention that kosher slaughter, which does not allow stunning, is not legal in New Zealand.

27. There is, of course, considerable debate concerning what the primary cause of this rise has been—whether, for example, soft drinks, fatty foods, white bread, or lack of exercise. We hope to address this debate elsewhere.

28. On lardo, see Cavanaugh 2005; on chitlins, see Poe 1999.

29. Flaps are importantly different from another fatty meat eaten in some Pacific Islands, namely Spam.™ First of all, Spam is too expensive to be widely eaten in places like Papua New Guinea. Indeed, even locally produced canned meat, such as corned beef, is losing out in many Pacific Islands (especially as re-frigeration becomes more available) to less-expensive, frozen meats, such as flaps. Moreover, as Lewis (2000) makes clear, in the Pacific Islands where Spam is eaten, it is assumed that white people positively value (or valued) it. It has, as well, be-come (especially in places like Hawaii) thoroughly traditionalized.

30. Fonua 2006.

31. Marks 2002.

32. Traders vehemently insist that they do not dump in the technical sense—and that their prices are entirely market-driven.

CHAPTER THREE

1. Hartsock (1985) argues that the Western market has always been dis-tinctly male. More recent analyses of the market concur. See, for example, Za-loom 2003 and 2004; Lynn 2004. Of course, the kind of masculinity valued by the purveyors of flaps is different from the fast-paced, in-your-face assertiveness of, for example, open-pit futures traders.

2. Maurer would probably draw the connection more closely. In his re-cently published book, he finds that "anthropology, like Islamic banking and alternative currencies, is a series of experiments . . . with the social significance and constitution of transactions" (2005, xv).

3. Lamb and mutton flaps are too low in value and too unpredictable in price to support a futures market. The obvious comparison is with pork bellies, which, at least in popular imagination, epitomize the speculative trading that constitutes commodity futures. Pork bellies can be the subject of commodity speculation because their supply, and the related demand for bacon, are not only relatively constant but can be tracked through established and publicly accessible indicators. Moreover, pork bellies (in large numbers) have substantial exchange value. Hence, because fluctuations in value are neither extreme nor random and transactions involve large sums, speculation about selling prices at particular times and places is both feasible and potentially lucrative. A lot of money can be made (and lost) by the numerous traders seeking accurately to predict minor rises

and falls in the market. We might point out that the meat traders with whom we worked, unlike those who trade in pork bellies, are concerned with getting a physical product from one place to another.

4. Firms are often looking for people who can do the job. One trader told us about an interview with such a prospect. "We were talking, and the guy mentioned that he had an interest in hunting, and so I asked him if he was going out that weekend. No, he was going to sell his grandfather's car. We talked about this, and he obviously had trading inclinations. He was good." Having trading inclinations means, of course, a willingness to take risks—although the independent meat traders we knew, unlike the currency traders studied by Zaloom (2003, 2004), did not use risk as a dominant trope to organize their lives. In fact, while acknowledging that theirs was a risky business, several told us that they were "risk averse": they worked hard to minimize risk.

5. *CL* means "chemically lean": thus "65% cl" would refer to meat with 35 percent fat.

6. Meat and Wool New Zealand 2003.

7. Meat and Wool New Zealand 2003, 28.

8. In one case, members of small firms united to try to negotiate lower shipping rates that would be more comparable to those given to the traders at the big processing companies.

9. These offices are also contexts for training. One trader described the training process thus:

> You train a guy mostly by just bringing him into the office. You don't give him a desk for the first three months. You tell him that if a seat is empty because someone is out, you can sit at his desk—but, when he comes back, you have to give it up. You also tell him that he has to listen to everything going on. But if someone says, get a cup of coffee, you get a cup of coffee. You do what you are told. Then, after three months or so, you ask him to do something like book the freight, and then everything starts coming together, and he makes his own contacts. At this point, you take him overseas and introduce him to clients. Eventually, he'll go by himself and be responsible for making his own deals.

10. Because the breast has the greater value, leg quarters are often leftovers.

11. Traders who do not sell into the Pacific Islands often characterize those who do as being willing to send anything, anywhere, in mixed containers—even, one joked, a transmission if a client wants it. We mentioned this to a trader who laughed and said, "Yes, I've actually sent up a Holden transmission." He went on to say that he would send up just about anything if he could make money on it. He was currently arranging to send some used, four-wheel-drive vehicles. The people in his firm who handled shipping were extremely good, and doing the paperwork for a mixed container was no problem for them.

12.   Pork imports are, for the most part, heavily tariffed to protect Papua New Guinea's own pig industry. Offal can be imported duty free because it is assumed that it will be reprocessed by a Papua New Guinea business into sausage and the like. Pig jowls, however, are being sold in Papua New Guinea as such—without reprocessing.

13.   Another innovation we learned about also involved moving quickly into shifting economic niches so as to seize temporary advantages. For instance, in December 2003, just as "mad cow" disease was reported in the United States, a New Zealand trader was entertaining a visiting Korean client. The client knew that Korea would immediately ban U.S. beef imports and that this might provide an opportunity for them both because it would create a demand in Korea for non-- U.S.-sourced beef intestines to be used in hot-pots and in barbequing. The United States had monopolized this trade—some ten thousand tons a year: its intestines were inexpensive to obtain and to process. Because of the availability of cheap water in the United States, processing plants could produce Grade A—fully flushed—intestines at a very good price. New Zealand had not even attempted to participate in this trade because its water was so expensive. However, with the United States (temporarily) out of the picture, New Zealand could perhaps move in with a less fully flushed product—a Grade B or Grade C. Recognizing this opportunity, the trader contacted the manager of a meat-processing firm with whom he had a good relationship. (In fact, he sent his son to apprentice with this manager before he allowed him to join his trading firm, believing that anyone selling meat should know his way around a carcass. He himself had "come up" in processing plants.) Together, the trader and manager quickly innovated by adapting a machine (flown in from the United States) that was used in hog processing. Using only minimal water, this machine cleaned the New Zealand beef intestines by running them through a kind of wringer that expelled most of their contents. The trader told us that, because he was "the first cab out of the rank," he got 90 percent of the Korean intestine market the first year. However, since the machine was readily available and adaptation straightforward, others immediately entered the field, and in the second year he got only 10 percent of this market. In telling us this story, the trader mentioned that this had been really enjoyable since he was able to articulate so well between his client and his processor—to the mutual advantage of all.

14.   Flaps are thus very different from branded and patented products such as Coca-Cola. See Foster 2008.

15.   In this sense, they are "hopeful," like Miyazaki's Japanese derivatives traders (2006), and involved in a moral project, like Maurer's Islamic bankers and alternative money users (2005).

16.   In this sense, we are reminded of Sahlins's discussion of Captain Cook as like "Adam Smith's global agent," committed to "the peaceful 'penetration' of

the marketplace: of commercial expansion, promising to bring civilization to the benighted and riches to the entire earth" (1985, 131).

17.   Some traders believe that Fiji could be a partial exception to this circumstance but for its recent history of political instability.

18.   The analogy is additionally interesting. If selling cars and selling parts of dead animals are activities that some disparage, this may encourage those who do so in two opposed ways: to create solidarity among all involved and to seek differentiation from the others by positioning themselves at the upper end of the market.

CHAPTER FOUR

1.   As of 1886, the northern half of what became the country of Papua New Guinea was a German colony, and the southern half was a British colony. In 1921, after World War I, the northern half—New Guinea—came under Australian administration, first as a League of Nations Mandated Territory and, then as a United Nations Trust Territory. In 1906, the southern half—Papua—though still formally controlled by Britain, also came under Australian administration. The two territories—New Guinea and Papua—were separately administered by Australia until 1942. Subsequently, Australia brought both under a single administration (although the United Nations retained some responsibility for the New Guinea portion). This condition prevailed until Papua New Guinea's independence as a single nation in 1975.

2.   See Finney 1971.

3.   The increasing consumption of lamb and mutton flaps in Papua New Guinea is documented by export figures from New Zealand and Australia, the predominant suppliers of sheep meat to this region. According to Meat and Wool New Zealand, exports of lamb and mutton flaps into Papua New Guinea increased from 4,480 tons in 1999 to 6,103 tons in 2005. Comparably, according to Meat and Livestock Australia, the export of flaps into Papua New Guinea increased from 6,257 tons in 1996 to 11,111 tons in 2005. The data concerning New Zealand were provided in an e-mail message received on May 2, 2006, from a representative of Meat and Wool New Zealand. The data concerning Australia were provided in an e-mail message received on May 15, 2006, from a representative of Meat and Livestock Australia.

4.   On the ways in which Papua New Guineans and others reconfigure the meaning and uses of Western commodities, see Carrier and Carrier 1989; Thomas 1991; and Sahlins 1992.

5.   On the ways in which one Papua New Guinean people view white men as borderline sociopaths, see Bashkow 2006.

6. Of course, those who did find work might disappoint as well. Consider the following translated letter from a young Wewak migrant, only sporadically working as a laborer, to his parents in Chambri, which illustrates both their expectation that he remit and his difficulty in doing so:

> Dear Mama and Daddy
> Hello and good night to both of you. It's been a very long time since I have written to you both. Also, I received the message you sent me. Concerning the money you want, I will send it in August of this year. About Christmas, I cannot say when or if I will come. But, I really mean that I will send the money to you, although I cannot say how much I will send. And don't think that I'll come for sure at Christmas. That's all now, except that I was happy to receive your message. Say a big hello to Timothy and Albert. So, that's all.

7. See Carrier and Carrier 1989 for an analysis of how remittances caused a cultural efflorescence by providing the commodities that were converted into ceremonial gifts in village contexts.

8. These must be taken as rough statistics; the accuracy of the census data collected in Papua New Guinea, given the illiteracy of many people, is questionable and certainly varies from region to region.

9. In 1987, 43 percent of the adult Chambri population over the age of seventeen lived away from Chambri Island; 15 percent of those away lived in Chambri Camp.

10. During the first six months of 1987, three Chambri were arrested for two separate thefts—one a robbery at knife point, the other a burglary—and three Chambri suffered attack: one rape, one stabbing, one death as a result of beating.

11. The women back home in the villages, upon hearing of this young woman's fears, denied that she would be in serious danger if she returned to Chambri. Many said that the real reason she and other young women remained in Wewak was that they were too lazy to fish and gather firewood. One told us resentfully, "They say we smell of fish; they like to walk around town smelling of perfume; they prefer to be supported by others rather than working hard themselves."

12. Many people throughout the world follow prescriptive marriage rules. In the case of the Chambri, a man is supposed marry his mother's brother's daughter or someone he calls mother's brother's daughter. In so doing, he will also marry someone from the moiety group opposite to his own.

13. For an accessible and compelling portrayal of how the promises of development have played out among one group of Highlanders living in the Mount Hagen area during the mid-1980s, see the film *Joe Leahy's Neighbours* (Connolly and Anderson 1988).

14. When Papua New Guinea became independent, the new government adopted a set of widely publicized "Eight Aims" that became its philosophical basis. One of these aims was to "create a more self-reliant economy, less dependent . . . on

imported goods and services and better able to meet the needs of its people through local production." The James Barnes factory was fostered to satisfy this aim by reducing imports and providing employment. The idea was to grow cattle in the Ramu Valley for the local production of canned corned beef. Unfortunately, the domestic cattle industry never proved sufficient to meet Barnes's needs, and the company relies heavily on imports.

15. Papua New Guinea has a heavily import-focused economy.

16. For a social impact study of this cannery, see Sullivan et al. 2003.

17. For an excellent survey of the literature about the nutritional health of Papua New Guineans, see Hughes 2003.

18. Roughly speaking, Papua New Guineans belong to two large and different genetic families: Austronesians and non-Austronesians. Austronesians are genetically related to Polynesians, who ostensibly possess "thrifty genes." (See chapter 1, note 39, for an elaboration and problematization of the thrifty gene hypothesis.) According to Sakaue and his colleagues, "Austronesian-speaking people in PNG have been reported to share the same genotype with Polynesians. Therefore, it is expected that the prevalence of obesity and type 2 diabetes will increase at least to the same extent as currently seen in Polynesians with westernization of their lifestyle" (Sakaue et al. 2003, 956).

19. These rates went up 21 percent and 17 percent, respectively. See Gibson and Rozelle 1998.

20. Saweri 2001.

21. Hodge, Dowse, and Zimmet 1996.

22. Saweri 2001, 151.

23. Muntwieler and Shelton 2001, as summarized in Saweri 2001, 157.

24. Gibson and Rozelle 1998; Gibson 2001.

25. Temu and Saweri 2001, 403.

26. Lamb tongues used to be plentiful throughout Papua New Guinea but are now rarely sold. The type preferred there, known as a "long cut" because it included the esophagus, could only be obtained by splitting the skull open. This was cost-effective while there was a European market for brains. When this market disappeared (given fears about mad cow disease and its possible analogues in sheep and other brains), it was no longer cost-effective to process tongues for the Papua New Guinea market. In fact, by 2006, tongues had tripled in price and were more expensive to buy from producers than some (lower-quality) lamb chops.

CHAPTER FIVE

1. See, especially, Pearson 1995.

2. Concerning the ritual of wrapping, see Carrier 1995.

3. Seneviratne 2001, 4.

4. Ipi 2002.

5. Jane Kelsey, a New Zealand scholar specializing in trade law, makes this argument. She believes that the ready import of such "fatty waste products" discourages local food production and thus fosters the "explicit links between dependence and [these] imported foods" (2004, 4).

6. *Post Courier*, October 27, 2005.

7. Daniel Kapi, as reported by O'Callaghan 1996.

8. See Poe 1999.

9. In an interesting discussion of what certain Papua New Guineans define as "white man's food," anthropologist Ira Bashkow writes that lamb and mutton flaps are a "racially ambiguous food." They are known to come from "white men's country." On they other hand, they resemble pork and have not been processed to the point that their "animal origin is no longer recognizable" (2006, 200–201).

10. Our excellent research assistants were Frances Akuani, Nellie Alman, Gende Louis Ambane, Ian N. Apeit, Rebecca Emori, Paula Gande, Kritoe Keleba, Dickson Mandengat, Joshua Meraveka, Alois Ralai, James Topo, and Malawa Wong.

11. In addition, students were asked to confirm by checking a box on the questionnaire "that the person knows that he/she does not have to answer any questions, but that help is very much appreciated."

12. They interviewed 65 from Madang, 63 from Mount Hagen, 62 from Gusap, 60 from Goroka, and 39 from Kerowagi. Fifteen were between 14 and 19; 51 were between 20 and 24; 58 were between 25 and 29; 51 were between 35 and 30; 58 were between 40 and 44; 27 were 45 or older; and the age of 1 was unknown.

13. Forty-seven sold flaps at markets; 25 were subsistence gardeners who occasionally sold vegetables at markets; 7 grew coffee; 7 owned trade stores; 6 sold betel nuts at markets; 2 sold used clothes at markets; 2 were pastors with small stipends; 2 worked occasionally as housegirls; 1 bought coffee; 1 repaired shoes on the street.

14. This figure includes 13 housewives, 9 students, and 2 whose occupations were unreported.

15. At the time of the interviews, a 20 kg carton of lamb and mutton flaps in Goroka varied in price from K102 to K110 (US$34–US$37), while a 1 kg package varied from K5.95 to K7.90 (US$2–US$2.60).

16. Concerning the continued value of pigs in one region of Papua New Guinea, see the film *Man Without Pigs*. It is about the return of historian John Waiko to his village, where he learns that having a Ph.D. does not trump having no pigs. See Owen 1990.

17. Rappaport 1968, 60.

18. Anthropologist Paige West reports that among Seventh-day Adventists in the Eastern Highlands Province, lamb and mutton flaps "totally replace pigs (and they do in brideprice, marriage, compensation and the like)" (personal communication via e-mail, May 28, 2006). Anthropologist George Westermark agrees, finding that in the Kainantu area, "Lamb flaps . . . were essential to ceremonies since so many people were Seventh-day Adventists, . . . [and] no food could be eaten from a mumu [an earth oven] where pig was included" (personal communication via e-mail, May 25, 2006).

19. A 10K loan for a period of less than two weeks would be repaid with 13K.

20. We were told that if the court were to release the money held in escrow, Mari had agreed to pay their creditors K1.50 for every K1.00 borrowed. Moreover, release of the money would not necessarily be the final word on which ethnic group actually owned the land.

21. We were in Madang when the decision about whether to release the sugar money from escrow prior to hearing the land case was to be made in court there. Many Mari had made the three-and-a-half-hour trip to learn the verdict. However (as seems quite typical according to newspaper accounts), the lawyer for one of the contesting groups had missed his plane out of Port Moresby, and so the case was postponed—initially for two weeks and subsequently repeatedly. Eventually, the case was heard. The court decided to divide the money in escrow among all of the disputing groups and to recognize the Mari as the official landowners after 2010. Both of these decisions are being appealed by one of the contestants and, as RSL's chief entomologist Lastus Kuniata put it, "there is now a lot of confusion" (personal communication via e-mail, January 8, 2008).

22. *Post Courier*, November 6, 2003.

23. See Saweri 2001.

24. We must qualify somewhat here. In our experience, when nonaffluent Papua New Guineans, whether rural or urban, had a personal connection with a politician such that they could make claims on him, then that politician's corpulence might be a respected sign of success. In the absence of such a connection, it was likely to arouse cynicism and fear.

25. Flaps are thus very different from, for example, the Atlantic bluefin tuna that Bestor (2001 and 2004) traces, which is an exquisite morsel for the hyperwealthy and refined.

CHAPTER SIX

1. Public debate about curtailing the trade is, however, recurrent. As this book goes to press, there has been a new flurry of discussion in Papua New Guinea's

national newspaper about whether flaps should be banned. Jamie Maxtone-Graham, who is a member of Parliament and cardiologist, was reported as planning to "introduce a bill into Parliament . . . banning the import and selling of lamb flaps, a cut of meat that is almost pure fat" (Ban Lamb Flaps 2009). Another physician, who is technical advisor for lifestyle disease at PNG's Department of Health, agreed with him in a letter entitled "Back MP's Efforts to Ban Lamb Flaps" (Vinit 2009). This was promptly qualified by yet another PNG physician in a letter entitled "Not All Metabolic Diseases Caused by Lamb Flaps" (Ongugo 2009). This flurry provoked a feature writer to retort that "I've heard that music before! . . . This issue has been making the rounds of Parliament for every term that you can remember. It seems that for want of something pressing to talk about in Parliament, some MP would come up with the idea of banning lamb flaps" (Meta 2009).

2. On the issue of the global regulation of drugs such as tobacco, see especially Reid 2005.

3. Martin 2007a.

4. National Food and Nutrition Centre 2007, 91.

5. National Food and Nutrition Centre 2007, 168.

6. See Cornelius et al. 2002.

7. Kumar 2000.

8. See Lawrence 2003 for an elaboration of such strategic formulations.

9. See especially Slatter 2003, 5.

10. The South Pacific Commission is charged with developing the technical, professional, scientific, and management capabilities of Pacific Island people so that they can "make and implement informed decisions about their future" (South Pacific Commission 2005).

11. Craig 1997.

12. Thompson, quoted in Choudry 2002.

13. Walsh and Mold 2003.

14. Cook 2004.

15. In 1999, Australia exported 872 tons of sheep meat (both lamb and mutton) to Fiji, none of which consisted of flaps.

16. Yet, several health professionals insisted that, before the ban, the country seemed awash in flaps. This appeared to be the case, no doubt, because flaps are conspicuous by virtue of their evident fattiness. However, we think this perception also may reflect their disproportionate presence in rural areas. The meat wholesalers who stock these areas are generally Indo-Fijians and therefore avoid carrying either beef or pork, lest they offend their Hindu and Moslem compatriots. Thus, in meeting the needs of rural markets for inexpensive meats, these wholesalers could most easily (and cheaply) supply low-value cuts of sheep meat—at the time, lamb and mutton flaps.

17. Parkinson 1999.

18. Vatucawaqa and Owen 2002; Vatucawaqa and Chand 2002.

19. Vatucawaqa 2002.

20. Kelsey 2004.

21. Karen Brison, personal communication.

22. The interviews were conducted by two social science students from the University of the South Pacific, Pateresio Nunu Polania and Patricia Matilda Bibi. Those they interviewed were selected from public places, relatively randomly.

23. The students also conducted forty-three interviews with people working directly with meat: butchers, owners of restaurants, and meat-counter attendants. Twenty-eight of these thought the ban was a good idea because flaps were low-quality, fatty, and had been dumped on Fiji. Eight disapproved of the ban because the market should dictate what was sold or not. And seven were ambivalent because flaps were unhealthful but were also popular and easy to sell. Interestingly, even those with a directly commercial engagement with meat shared the perspectives of ordinary citizens.

24. Sponsoring organizations include the Wellcome Trust (an independent charity devoted to promoting human and animal health based in the United Kingdom), the Health Resource Council of New Zealand, the National Health and Medical Research Council of Australia, and the World Health Organization (WHO).

25. When we met with him in his Auckland office, he shared with us the powerpoint presentation he used to explain OPIC to government officials. See Scragg 2006.

26. Of the 1,429 Pacific Islanders studied in New Zealand, 52 percent were of Samoan origin, 21 percent of Tongan origin, 14 percent of Cook Island origin, 7 percent of Niuean origin, 2 percent of Tokelauan origin, 2 percent of Fijian origin; and 2 percent were designated "other." According to the official report, "one-third of Pacific boys and girls were overweight and a further 26% of the boys and 31% of the girls were obese. . . . Only just over one half of the Pacific children usually had something to eat before they left home in the morning for school. Over 13% of Pacific children brought most of the food they consumed at school from the canteen or tuckshop." The report presents the data concerning Maori and NZEO children in New Zealand somewhat differently. Concerning Maori children, it states that "41% . . . were either overweight or obese, and this was a particular concern among girls (47%)"; that "66% of Maori girls and 75% of Maori boys usually had something to eat before they left home in the morning for school"; and that "about three out of four children brought most of the food they consumed at school from home." Concerning NZEO children, it states that "three-quarters . . . had a weight that was within an acceptable limit in relation

to their height"; that "94% of NZEO boys and 88% of NZEO girls usually had something to eat before they left home in the morning for school;" and that "over 90% of NZEO children brought most of the food they consumed at school from home" (New Zealand Ministry of Health 2003).

27. For an excellent review article that includes a comprehensive bibliography concerning the differences between anthropology and epidemiology, see DiGiacomo 1999. For a somewhat less critical view, see Trostle and Sommerfeld 1996; and Trostle 2005.

28. Schultz et al. 2006, 5.

29. In this regard, a recent article from the BBC news (2008) cited a study at the University of Minnesota that provided a different narrative of why kids who ate breakfast at home remained leaner than those who did not (although it still leaves us with many questions). Interestingly, the breakfast-eaters consumed more calories, but "did more to burn those off, and that may be because those who ate breakfast at home did not feel so lethargic."

30. Schultz et al. 2006, 8.

31. In fact, an earlier draft of the report relates (to summarize) that the majority of indigenous Fijian males had breakfast at home regularly, and eight stated that breakfast was their biggest/most important meal of the day; the majority of Indo-Fijian males had breakfast regularly, and four stated that breakfast was the biggest/most important meal of the day; more than half of the indigenous Fijian females (thirteen) often skipped breakfast, but four stated that breakfast was their biggest/most important meal of the day; the majority of Indo-Fijian females (sixteen) skipped breakfast regularly, but seven reported that breakfast was the biggest/most important meal of the day, and nine said that their parents forced them to eat breakfast (Schultz et al. 2006 11).

32. Becker 1995, 84.

33. Focus 1999.

34. Focus 1999.

35. See Becker, Gilman, and Burwell 2005 for the complete analysis. Among the interventions Becker suggests are "psychoeducational information about the psychological risks associated with binging, purging, and self-starvation as well as media literacy programs that instruct youth in critical and informed viewing of televised programming and commercials" (2004, 556).

36. As background to the task of tackling obesity in the Pacific, the OPIC team endorses the following excerpt from the report, *Obesity in the Pacific: Too Big to Ignore* (Gill et al. 2002): "An effective response to obesity faces many barriers. Culturally, large physical size is considered a mark of beauty and social status in many Pacific Island countries. At a community and policy-making level, there is resistance to the view that obesity is a health problem. Many

Pacific Island countries and territories depend on imported food, with commercial interests more likely to favour imports of high-fat, energy-dense foods. As food preferences among consumers in the Pacific change, imported and convenience food is afforded higher status. High rates of violence and crime reduce the opportunities for outdoor physical activity. For islands in transition, the inevitable growth in the use of modern technology sharply reduces physical activity and thus energy expenditure, adding to the problems created by the increase in sedentary occupations in urban areas of the Pacific region" (Commonwealth Secretariat 2006). This is a more complex perspective than the one it actually puts into operation.

37. National Health Promotion Council 2006, 5. In order to increase control and improve health, the country had been already divided into four districts and these into 272 self-designated "settings," such as villages, schools, markets, ports, towns, workplaces, and hotels—places where people live work, play, and interact daily. Inhabitants of each setting were to commit to an action plan—such as building a certain number of latrines, increasing the rates of breastfeeding, or reducing the use of alcohol and drugs by youth. Small amounts of money might be allocated to get plans started. Modular courses were provided by members of the Community Organization Development Committee (within the National Health Promotion Council) to teach people to evaluate their successes and failures: to help them monitor, build capacity, and achieve milestones. By implication, those involved assumed responsibility if goals were not met. At the meeting of the National Health Council we attended, those in charge of establishing and representing settings within districts enumerated the challenges they faced and the objectives they achieved—and were questioned about the former and congratulated for the latter. Why had this district lagged behind the others in establishing new settings? Why had a clean water supply not been made a priority as the people had requested? What might be learned from the success of one setting in reducing drinking by youth?

38. National Health Promotion Council 2006, 5.

39. National Health Promotion Council 2006, 11.

40. National Health Promotion Council 2006, 10. The international standards cited in the policy are those of the Codex Alimentarius, the World Trade Organization, and the World Health Organization.

41. Asian Development Bank 2005.

42. *Povi* means "cow" in Samoan; *pulu* means "cow" in Tongan; *masima* means "salt" in both languages.

43. Meat and Wool New Zealand subsequently produced a widely distributed poster—we saw it in butcher shops in South Auckland (where Pacific Islanders often live)—advising that *povi/pulu masima* should be boiled in water

that was changed two to three times; that all the fat should be trimmed from it before it was cooked; and that it should be served with plenty of colorful vegetables.

44. Heart Foundation of New Zealand 2004.

45. Lawrence and Swinburn 2004, 2.

46. Evans 1999, 138.

47. Places that rely on remittances from abroad are especially vulnerable to economic downturns in the countries where remitters have been working.

48. See Kingdom of Tonga Statistics Department 2002, 12.

49. During fieldwork in Tonga in 2008, anthropologist Niko Besnier discovered that flaps cost T$7/kg, while *pulu masima* cost T$14/kg (e-mail communication, February 11, 2008).

50. Kentucky Fried Chicken pieces are brought into the country as gifts to family and others. And, while there are no KFC (or other big-name, fast-food) outlets in Tonga, local fried chicken imitations are also referred to as KFC (Niko Besnier, e-mail communication, February 26, 2008).

51. Anthropologist Niko Besnier explained in a personal communication that the image of dumping recurs in other food-focused areas in Tonga "such as the import of past-due-date processed food like canned vegetables and juices and junk-food items like snacks ('Twisties')" (e-mail message, February 11, 2008). Of the items understood as substandard, the most objectionable would appear to be ones that those in the exporting countries would reject for themselves.

52. See Marshall 2004 for a discussion of turkey tails in Micronesia.

53. Interestingly, Samoa banned the import of turkey tails in 2007. This Pacific Island country is, however, under the direct influence of the United States.

CONCLUSION

1. New Zealand Joint Agency Report 2007.

2. According to the report, 34 percent went to China and 37 percent to the rest of the world.

3. New Zealand Joint Agency Report 2007, 9.

4. New Zealand Health Committee 2007, 31.

5. This minority response was that of members of the principal opposition party, the National Party.

6. New Zealand Health Committee 2007, 35.

7. The New Zealand Government is composed of the prime minister and the Cabinet. At the time that "Inquiry into Obesity and Type 2 Diabetes in New

Zealand" was released, the prime minister, Helen Clark, and all but one minister in her Cabinet, were members of the Labour Party. Thus, the government rejected a recommendation written by a committee largely composed of members of its own party or coalition members.

8. New Zealand Government 2007, 23.

9. Anthropologist Niko Besnier points out in a personal communication that this CNN characterization of Tonga is poorly informed since "coconut flesh is hardly a 'staple' in Tonga, and Tongans rarely eat it" (e-mail message, February 11, 2008).

10. Fonua 2006.

11. These calculations are based upon statistics provided in Swinburn 2004. Again, we have no independent verification that this woman was eating this amount, although we have no doubt that she was eating a lot.

12. Yamamoto, n.d.

13. In this regard, the privileged are unlike the many other Pacific Island peoples who, as the 1997 South Pacific Consumer Protection Programme we quoted in chapter 1 suggests, "have a limited choice in the market place because [they] have limited cash to buy food," a point we will return to.

14. Although the king is known to have had obesity-related cardiovascular problems, including diabetes, the cause of his death has not, by virtue of his sacredness, been officially revealed.

15. It would be a major accomplishment for someone accustomed to eating a liter of ice cream daily as a snack (together with either six pancakes or half a cake—not to mention the flaps!) to sustain the frugality of this diet through the loss of, perhaps, a hundred pounds.

16. Yamamoto, n.d.

17. New Zealand National Party 2005.

18. New Zealand Health Committee 2007, 35.

19. This quotation seems to have originated in Evelyn Hall's 1906 summary of Voltaire's ideas. Hall wrote under the pseudonym of Stephen Tallentyre.

20. Concerning these cultural standards as they played out in the life of the king of Tonga, anthropologist Niko Besnier conveyed the following to us in an e-mail message on January 10, 2008:

> [In Tonga] a seated body that looks like a pyramid indexes high status. Even the heads of the high ranking in Tonga have this odd shape that makes them look like it is continuous with the rest of the body, and people pick up on this feature to identify potential kinship ties to the high ranking. . . . In Taufa'ahau IV's case, I think many other factors came into play: constant feeding at obligatory feasts, . . . constant stream of food prestations up the social pyramid, barely being allowed to place one foot in front of the other, and probably having little interest in moving his body until he realized half-way through his life that he had to.

21. In fact, the king died at the age of eighty-eight. Indeed, according to 2005 data collected by the World Health Organization (WHO), he lived sixteen years longer than the average Tongan man. That being said, like many Tongans, he had been in ill health for quite some time prior to his death. He also lived longer than most Fijians and Papua New Guineans. According to 2002 data collected by the WHO, the life expectancy for the average Fijian man is sixty-six; for the average Papua New Guinean man, it is fifty-nine. See World Health Organization 2007.

22. Center for Consumer Freedom, n.d.a.

23. Center for Consumer Freedom, n.d.a.

24. Center for Consumer freedom, n.d.b. The cartoon appeared on the Center for Consumer Freedom's Web site: http://www.consumerfreedom.com/cartoons.cfm/page/9.

25. Texas Association for School Nutrition 2005.

26. This article appeared in Andrew Breitbart's online news site; see Breitbart 2008.

27. Interestingly, a report on a National Public Radio broadcast on January 5, 2008, about the new bans included a French commentator who bemoaned the new labels mandated to appear on French wine indicating that pregnant women should not consume alcoholic beverages. He described wine as a "totem" for the French, as an icon of French identity, arguing that it should not be regulated without protest. See Beardsley 2008.

28. We should point out that advocates of gun control in the United States also hear these arguments frequently.

29. Schlosser 2002; Pollan 2006.

30. Spurlock 2004.

31. See Martin 2007b.

32. Goizueta, quoted in Foster 2008, 65 and 66.

33. Foster 2002, 12.

34. Geographer Aaron Bobrow-Strain describes such a politics of personal consumption this way: "Today's food writers seem unwilling or unable to imagine political change occurring through anything but the reasoned, rational, consumer choices of an informed population, a political vision nicely summarized in Eric Schlosser's blurb on *Omnivore's Dilemma*: 'What should you eat? Michael Pollan addresses that fundamental question with great wit and intelligence. . . . Eating well, he finds, can be a pleasurable way to change the world'" (2007, 50).

35. Pollan's actual words are, "Eat food. Not too much. Mostly plants" (2008, 1).

36. Also, concerning national responses to eating stigmatized foods, consider the following 2006 news item from the New Zealand press at the time of our research:

Kenya dismissed as "culturally insulting" Tuesday an offer of powdered dog food to feed starving children reportedly made by the founder of a canine biscuit company in New Zealand.

"Kenyan kids are not so desperate as to eat dog food," Kenya government spokesman Alfred Mutua told Reuters in response to a front-page story in the East African country's leading daily" (Reuters 2006).

37. Templeton 2008.

38. For the ways in which McDonald's restaurants shape their modernist promise so as to fit different sociocultural contexts, see Watson 1997.

References

Abumrad, Nadia. 2005. CD36 May Determine Our Desire for Dietary Fats. *Journal of Clinical Investigation* 115:2965–67.

Aiello, Leslie, and Peter Wheeler. 1995. The Expensive Tissue Hypothesis: The Brain and the Digestive System in Human and Primate Evolution. *Current Anthropology* 36: 199–222.

Altucher, James. 2007. The Obesity Index. Available online at the Forbes Web site: http://www.forbes.com/investingideas/2007/04/16/nutrisystem -herbalife-obesity-pf-ii-in_ja_0416soapbox_inl.html (accessed June 3, 2007).

Anderson, Jan. 2004. Dairy Deregulation in Northern Queensland: The End of Traditional Farming? *Anthropological Forum* 14:269–82.

Asian Development Bank. 2005. Fiji Economy to Face Daunting Challenges Both in Domestic and External Fronts. Available online at http://www.adb.org/Documents/News/2005/nr2005047.asp (accessed August 5, 2007).

Australian Bureau of Agricultural Resources and Economics and the New Zealand Ministry of Agriculture and Forestry. 2006. *Agricultural Economies of Australia and New Zealand: Past, Present, Future*. Report to the Governments of Australia and New Zealand. Canberra: National Capital Printing.

Ban Lamb Flaps. 2009. Available online at http://www.thenational.com.pg/031609/nation31.php (accessed on April 11, 2009).

Barbecue Lamb Belly the Slow Way. n.d. Available online at http://www.vital.org.nzbarbecue-lamb.html (accessed on March, 11, 2006).

Barrett, James. 1987. *Work and Community in the Jungle: Chicago's Packinghouse Workers, 1894–1922*. Urbana: University of Illinois Press.

Bashkow, Ira. 2006. *The Meaning of Whitemen: Race and Modernity in the Orokaiva Cultural World*. Chicago: University of Chicago Press.

Baudrillard, Jean. 1981. *For a Critique of the Political Economy of the Sign*. New York: Telos Press.

BBC News. 2008. Breakfast "Keeps Teenagers Lean." Available online at http://newsvote.bbc.co.uk/mpapps/pagetools/print/news.bbc.co.uk/2/hi/health/7275554.stm (accessed on March 6, 2008).

Beardsley, Eleanor. 2008. Warning Labels Mandated for Wine Bottles in France. Available online at http://www.npr.org/templates/story/story.php?storyId = 17869405 (accessed on January 6, 2008).

Becker, Anne. 1995. *Body, Self, and Society: The View from Fiji*. Philadelphia: University of Philadelphia Press.

———. 2004. Television, Disordered Eating, and Young Women in Fiji: Negotiating Body Image and Identity During Rapid Social Change. *Culture, Medicine and Psychiatry* 28: 533–59.

Becker, Anne, Stephen Gilman, and Rebecca Burwell. 2005. Changes in Prevalence of Overweight and in Body Image among Fijian Women between 1989 and 1998. *Obesity Research* 13:110–17.

Bestor, Theodore. 2001. Supply-Side Sushi: Commodity, Market and the Global City. *American Anthropologist* 103:76–95.

———. 2004. *Tsukiji: The Fish Market at the Center of the World*. Berkeley and Los Angeles: University of California Press.

Bird, Graham, and Lee Norris. 2006. Temporary Migrant Workers: The Challenge for the AMIEU. Available online at http://www.amieu.asn.au/printout.php?recid = 120 (accessed on May 6, 2007).

Blundell, J. E., and J. I. MacDiarmid. 1997. Fat as a Risk Factor for Overconsumption. *Journal of the American Dietetics Association* 97 (supp. 7): 63–69.

Bobrow-Strain, Aaron. 2007. Kills a Body Twelve Ways: Bread Fear and the Politics of "What to Eat?" *Gastronomica* 7:45–52.

Bonanno, Alessandro. 2004. Globalization, Transnational Corporations, the State and Democracy. *International Journal of the Sociology of Agriculture and Food* 12:37–48.

Brandt, Deborah. 2002. *Tangled Routes: Women, Work and Globalization on the Tomato Trail.* Lanham, PA: Rowman and Littlefield.

Breitbart, Andrew. 2008. Europeans Chafe under New Year "Nanny State" Laws. Available online at http://www.breitbart.com/print.php?id = 080103055145.2hj5ecot&show_article = 1 (accessed January 3, 2008).

Bruni, Frank. 2007. Fat, Glorious Fat, Moves to the Center of the Plate. Available online at http://www.nytimes.com/2007/06/13/dining/13glut.html?_r = 1& scp = 2&sq = Bruni+Fat+glorious+Fat&oref = slogin (accessed June 13, 2007).

Burch, David, Jasper Goss, Geoffrey Lawrence, and Roy Rickson. 1999. The Global Restructuring of Food and Agriculture: Contingencies and Parallels in Australia and New Zealand. *Rural Sociology* 64:179–85.

Calder, Mick, and Janet Tyson. 1999. *Meat Acts.* Wellington: New Zealand Meat Board.

Callon, Michel, Cécile Meadel, and Vololona Rabehariosa. 2002. The Economy of Qualities. *Economy and Society* 31:194–217.

Carrier, James. 1995. *Gifts and Commodities: Exchange and Western Capitalism since 1700.* London: Routledge.

Carrier, James, and Achsah Carrier. 1989. *Wage, Trade, and Exchange in Melanesia: A Manus Society in the Modern State.* Berkeley and Los Angeles: University of California Press.

Cavanaugh, Jillian. 2005. Lard. In *Fat: The Anthropology of an Obsession*, ed Don Kulick and Anne Meneley, 139–52. New York: Penguin.

Center for Consumer Freedom. n.d.a. About Us. Available online at http://www.consumerfreedom.com/about.cfm (accessed on January 4, 2008).

———. n.d.b. Cartoons. Available online at http://www.consumerfreedom.com/cartoons.cfm (accessed on January 4, 2008).

Choudry, Aziz. 2002. Killing Me Softly. Available online at http://sydney.indymedia.org/print.php3?article_id = 17964 (accessed on August 5, 2003).

Commonwealth Secretariat. 2006. Obesity Prevention in Communities (OPIC). Available online at http://www.thecommonwealth.org/Shared_ASP_Files/UploadedFiles/E7445AEF-23E9-4FAC-B72D-8E5E5D54DA40_opic.pdf (accessed on July 27, 2007).

Conklin, Beth. 2001. *Consuming Grief: Compassionate Cannibalism in an Amazonian Society.* Austin: University of Texas Press.

Connolly, Bob, and Robin Anderson. 1988. *Joe Leahy's Neighbours.* Videorecording. Watertown, MA: Documentary Educational Resources.

Cook, Ian. 2004. Follow the Thing: Papaya. *Antipode* 36:642–64.

Cook, Stephen. 2004. Overstayer Abuses NZ Lifeline. Available online at http://www.businessherald.co.nz/print.cfm?objectid = 3577618 (accessed on October 17).

Cornelius, Margaret, Maximilliam Decourten, Jan Pryor, Sala, Saketa, Temo Waqanivalu, Apa Leqeretabua, and Elaine Chung. 2002. *Fiji Non-Communicable Diseases (NCD) Steps Survey.* Suva: Ministry of Health.

Coyne, Terry. 2000. *Lifestyle Diseases in Pacific Communities.* Noumea: Secretariat of the Pacific Community.

Craig, Cheryl. 1997. Unpublished letter sent to Robert Hughes by the General Manager of International Services at the New Zealand Meat Producers Board.

Curtis, Michael. 2004. The Obesity Epidemic in the Pacific. *Journal of Development and Social Transformation* 1:37–42.

Dahlberg, Frances, ed. 1981. *Woman the Gatherer.* New Haven, CT: Yale University Press.

Diabetes Genetics Initiative of the Broad Institute of Harvard and MIT, Lund University, and Novartis Institutes for BioMedical Research. 2007. Genome-Wide Association Analysis Identifies Loci for Type 2 Diabetes and Triglyceride Levels. *Science* 316:1331–36.

DiGiacomo, Susan. 1999. Can There Be a "Cultural Epidemiology"? *Medical Anthropology Quarterly* 13:436–57.

Dixon, Janet. 2002. *The Changing Chicken: Chooks, Cooks, and Culinary Culture.* Sydney: University of New South Wales Press.

Dominguez-Rodrigo, Manuel. 1997. Meat-Eating by Early Hominids at the FLK 22 *Zinjanthropus* Site, Olduvai Gorge (Tanzania): An Experimental Approach Using Cut-Mark Data. *Journal of Human Evolution* 33: 669–90.

Drewnowski, Adam. 1999. Fat and Sugar in the Global Diet: Dietary Diversity in the Nutrition Transition. In *Food in Global History*, ed. Raymond Grew, 194–206. Boulder, CO: Westview Press.

Eaton, S. Boyd, and Marjorie Shostak. 1986. Fat Tooth Blues. *Natural History* 95:8–11.

Eaton, S. Boyd, Steve Eaton, and Melvin Konner. 1997. Paleolithic Nutrition Revisited: A Twelve-Year Retrospective on Its Nature and Implications. *European Journal of Clinical Nutrition* 51: 207–16.

Emergency Response and Research Institute. 1991. Available online at http://www.emergency.com/nc-fire.htm (accessed on November 3, 2006).

Errington, Frederick, and Deborah Gewertz. 1987. *Cultural Alternatives and a Feminist Anthropology.* Cambridge: Cambridge University Press.

———. 2004. *Yali's Question: Sugar, Culture, and History.* Chicago: University of Chicago Press.

Ettlinger, Steve. 2007. What Twinkies Can Teach Us. *Daily Hampshire Gazette*, July 23, A6.

Evans, Mike. 1999. Is Tonga's MIRAB Economy Sustainable? *Pacific Studies* 22: 137–166.

Evans, Mike, Robert Sinclair, Caroline Fusimalohi, and Viliami Liava'a. 2001. Globalization, Diet, and Health: An Example from Tonga. *Bulletin of the World Health Organization* 79: 856–62.

Evans, Mike, Robert Sinclair, Caroline Fusimalohi, Viliami Liava'a, and Milton Freedman. 2003. Consumption of Traditional Versus Imported Foods in Tonga: Implications for Programs Designed to Reduce Diet-Related Non-Communicable Diseases in Developing Countries. *Ecology of Food and Nutrition* 42:153–76.

Feeley-Harnik, Gillian. 1981. *The Lord's Table*. Washington, DC: Smithsonian Institution Press.

Ferreira, Mariana, and Gretchen Lang. 2006. Introduction: Deconstructing Diabetes. In *Indigenous Peoples and Diabetes Community Empowerment and Wellness*, ed. Mariana Ferreira and Gretchen Lang, 3–32. Durham, NC: Carolina Academic Press.

Fiddes, Nick. 1991. *Meat, a Natural Symbol*. London: Routledge.

Finney, Ben. 1971. Bigfellow Man Bilong Business in New Guinea. In *Melanesia*, ed. L. L. Langness and John Weschler, 315–32. Scranton, PA: Chandler.

Fischer, Edward, and Peter Benson. 2006. *Broccoli and Desire: Global Connections and Maya Struggles in Postwar Guatemala*. Stanford, CA: Stanford University Press.

Fletcher, Anthony. 2005. Fat Taste Receptor Discovery Could Influence Food Formulation. Available online at http://www.meatprocess.com/news/ng .asp?n = 63700-taste-fat-obesity (accessed on December 11, 2006).

Focus. 1999. Shape Rise in Disordered Eating in Fiji Follows Arrival of Western TV. Available online at http://focus.hms.harvard.edu/1999/May28_1999/soc .html (accessed on June 24, 2005).

Foley, Robert. 2001. The Evolutionary Consequences of Increased Carnivory in Hominids. In *Meat-Eating and Human Evolution*, ed. Craig Stanford and Henry Bunn, 305–31. Oxford: Oxford University Press.

Foley, Robert, and Phyllis Lee. 1991. Ecology and Energetics of Encephalization in Hominid Evolution. *Philosophical Transactions of the Royal Society* 334:223–32.

Fonua, Pesi. 2006. Taufa'ahau Tupou IV, Tonga King 41 Years. Available online at http://www.washingtonpost.com/wp-dyn/content/article/2006/09/10/ AR2006091000902.html (accessed on November 3, 2006).

Foster, Robert. 2002. *Materializing the Nation: Commodities, Consumption and Media in Papua New Guinea*. Bloomington: Indiana University Press.

———. 2006. Tracking Globalization. In *Handbook of Material Culture,* ed. Christopher Tilley, Webb Keane, Susanne Küchler, Mike Rowlands, and Patricia Spyer, 285–302. London: Sage.

———. 2008. *Coca-Globalization: Following Soft Drinks from New York to New Guinea.* New York: Palgrave Macmillan.

Freidberg, Susanne. 2004. *French Beans and Food Scares: Culture and Commerce in an Anxious Age.* Oxford: Oxford University Press.

Geertz, Clifford. 1973. Deep Play: Notes on the Balinese Cock Fight. In *The Interpretation of Cultures,* ed. Clifford Geertz, 412–53. New York: Basic Books.

Gewertz, Deborah, and Frederick Errington. 1991. *Twisted Histories, Altered Contexts: Representing the Chambri in a World System.* Cambridge: Cambridge University Press.

———. 1999. *Emerging Class in Papua New Guinea: The Telling of Difference.* Cambridge: Cambridge University Press.

———. 2007. The Alimentary Forms of the Global Life. *American Anthropologist* 109:496–508.

Gibson, John. 2001. The Nutritional Status of PNG's Population. In *Food Security for Papua New Guinea,* ed. R. Michael Bourke, Matthew Allen and J.G. Salisbury, 407–13. Canberra: Australian Centre for international Agricultural Research.

Gibson, John, and Scott Rozelle. 1998. *Results of the Household Survey Component of the 1996 Poverty Assessment for PNG.* Report Submitted to the World Bank, Washington, DC.

Gill, Tim, Robert Hughes, Jimaima Tunidau-Schultz, Chizuru Nishida, Gauden Galea, and Tommasso Cavalli-Sforza. 2002. *Obesity in the Pacific: Too Big to Ignore.* Noumea: Secretariat of the Pacific Community.

Hannerz, Ulf. 1992. The Global Ecumene as a Network of Networks. In *Conceptualizing Society,* ed. A. Kuper, 34–56. London: Routledge.

Harris, David. 2003. Agricultural Policy Reform and Industry Adjustment: Some Recent Experience in Australia. Paper presented at the International Agricultural Policy Reform and Adjustment Project (IAPRAP) workshop entitled Policy Reform and Adjustment, Imperial College London, Wye Campus.

Harris, David, and Allan Rae. 2006. Agricultural Policy Reform and Industry Adjustment in Australia and New Zealand. In *Policy Reform and Adjustment in the Agricultural Sectors of Developed Countries,* ed. David Blandford and Berkeley Hill, 83–103. Wallingford, UK: CAB International Publishing.

Harris, Marvin. 1985. *Good to Eat: Riddles of Food and Culture.* New York: Simon and Schuster.

Hart, Donna, and Robert Sussman. 2005. *Man the Hunted: Primates, Predators and Human Evolution.* New York: Westview Press.

Hartsock, Nancy. 1985. Exchange Theory: Critique from a Feminist Perspective. In *Current Perspectives in Social Theory*, ed. Scott McNall, 57–70. Greenwich, CT: JAI Press.

Hayes, Brian. 2005. *Infrastructure: The Book of Everything for the Industrial Landscape*. New York: W. W. Norton.

Hayman, Kamala. 2006. The Changing Face of a Town. *Christchurch Press*, Wednesday, March 22, n.p.

Heart Foundation of New Zealand. 2004. *Report of the Povi/Pulu Masima Study*. Auckland: Heart Foundation of New Zealand.

Heatherington, M., and B. Rolls. 1996. Sensory-Specific Satiety. In *Why We Eat What We Eat*, ed. E. Capaldu, 267–90. Washington, DC: American Psychological Association.

Herness, M. Scott, and Timothy Gilbertson. 1999. Cellular Mechanisms of Taste Transduction. *Annual Review of Physiology* 61:873–900.

Hodge, Allison, Gary Dowse, and Paul Zimmet. 1996. Obesity in Pacific Populations. *Pacific Health Dialog* 3:77–86.

Holland, Anna. 2005. Dogs Dietary Needs Similar to Top Athletes. *New Zealand Farmers Weekly*, Available online at http://www.country-wide.co.nz/a-man/view.php (accessed on March 5, 2006).

Hone, Philip, and Henry Haszler. 2004. Trends in Obesity in Fiji. Unpublished research paper funded by the Australian Centre for International Agricultural Research.

Horowitz, Roger. 1997. *Negro and White, Unite and Fight: A Social History of Industrial Unionism in Meatpacking, 1930–90*. Champaign: University of Illinois Press

———. 2005. *Putting Meat on the American Table: Taste, Technology, Transformation*. Baltimore, MD: Johns Hopkins University Press.

Hughes, Robert. 2001. *Nutrition in Papua New Guinea: Literature Review Carried Out for the PNG Health Services Support Program*. Unpublished Report. Port Moresby: PNG Health Services Support Program.

———. 2003. *Diet, Food Supply and Obesity in the Pacific*. Geneva: World Health Organization.

Hughes, Robert, and Mark Lawrence. 2005. Globalisation, Food and Health in Pacific Island Countries. *Asia Pacific Journal of Clinical Nutrition* 14:298–306.

Industry Commission. 1994. *Meat Processing*. Melbourne: Australian Government Publishing Service.

Ipi, Yarapaki. 2002. Let's Do Something about the Sliding Kina! Available online at http://www.thenational.com.pg/1113/opinion10.htm (accessed on October 8, 2003).

Jansen, A. A. J., Susan Parkinson, and A. F. S. Robertson. 1990. *Food and Nutrition in Fiji: A Historical Review*. Suva: University of the South Pacific.

Kahn, Mirian. 1986. *Always Hungry, Never Greedy: Food and Expression of Gender in a Melanesian Society.* Cambridge: Cambridge University Press.

Kelsey, Jane. 2004. Acceding Countries as Pawns in a Power Play: A Case Study of the Pacific Islands. Paper presented at the WTO. Public Symposium, Multilateralism at the Crossroads. Geneva, May 27.

Kingdom of Tonga Statistics Department. 2002. *Report on the Household Income and Expenditure Survey.* Available online at http://www.spc.int/prism/country/to/stats/pdfs/HIES/HIES_2000_01.pdf (accessed February 23, 2003).

Kneen, Brewster. 1999. Restructuring Food for Corporate Profit: The Corporate Genetics of Cargill and Monsanto. *Agriculture and Human Values* 16:161–67.

Kumar, A. 2000. Legal Document No. 14. Archived material, Ministry of Commerce, Business Development and Investment, Suva, Fiji.

Lako, Jimaima, and Van Chuyen Nguyen. 2001. Dietary Patterns and Risk Factors in Diabetes Mellitus among Urban Indigenous Women in Fiji. *Asia Pacific Journal of Clinical Nutrition* 10:88–193.

Larsen, Clark Spencer. 2003. Animal Source Foods and Human Health During Evolution. *Journal of Nutrition* 133 (11, supp. 2): 3893S–97S.

Laugerette, Fabienne, Patricia Passilly-Degrace, Bruno Patris, Isabelle Niot, Maria Febbraio, Jeani Pierre Montmayeur, and Phillipe Besnard. 2005. CD36 Involvement in Orosensory Detection of Dietary Lipids, Spontaneous Fat Preference, and Digestive Secretions. *Journal of Clinical Investigation* 115:3177–84.

Lawrence, Geoffrey. 1987. *Capitalism and the Countryside: The Rural Crisis in Australia.* Sydney: Pluto Press.

————. 1999. Agri-Food Restructuring: A Synthesis of Recent Australian Research. *Rural Sociology* 64:186–202.

Lawrence, Geoffrey, and Frank Vanclay. 1994. Agricultural Change in the Semiperiphery: The Murray-Darling Basin, Australia. In *The Global Restructuring of Agro-Food Systems,* ed. Philip McMichael, 76–103. Ithaca, NY: Cornell University Press.

Lawrence, Mark. 2003. *Using Domestic Law in the Fight Against Obesity.* Geneva: World Health Organization.

Lawrence, Mark, and Boyd Swinburn. 2004. *The Food and Nutrition System in Tonga: The Roles and Functions of Relevant Jurisdictions with Respect to the Development and Implementation of Appropriate Legislative Provisions and Related Capacity-building Requirements.* Technical Report. Nuku'alofa, Tonga: Government of Tonga.

Leach, Edmund. 1972. Anthropological Aspects of Language: Animal Categories and Verbal Abuse. In *Mythology,* ed. Pierre Maranda, 39–76. Harmondsworth, UK: Penguin.

Lee, Richard, and Irven Devore, eds. 1968. *Man the Hunter.* Chicago: Aldine.

Leonard, William. 2002. Dietary Change Was a Driving Force in Human Evolution. *Scientific American* 288:63–71.

Lewis, George. 2000. From Minnesota Fat to Seoul Food: Spam in America and the Pacific Rim. *Journal of Popular Culture* 34: 83–105.

Llambi, Luis. 1993. Global Agro-Food Restructuring: The Role of Transnational Corporations and Nation-States. *International Journal for the Sociology of Agriculture and Food* 3:19–38.

Lynn, Cari. 2004. *Leg the Spread: A Woman's Adventures Inside the Trillion-Dollar Boys' Club of Commodity Trading.* New York: Broadway Books.

Mahler, Sarah. 1995. *American Dreaming.* Princeton, NJ: Princeton University Press.

Marcus, George. 1995. Ethnography in/of the World System. *Annual Review of Anthropology* 24:95–117.

Marks, Kathy. 2002. Pacific Islanders' Fatal Diet Blamed on Kiwi Exports. Available online at http://www.findarticles.com/p/articles/mi_qn4158/is_20020324/ai_n12597020 (accessed on October 18, 2006).

Marshall, Mac. 2004. *Namoluk Beyond the Reef.* Boulder, CO: Westview Press.

Martin, Andrew. 2007a. Will Diners Still Swallow This? Available online at http://select.nytimes.com/search/restricted/article?res = F30A16FB3E540C768EDDAA0894DF404482 (accessed on March 25, 2007).

———. 2007b. Did McDonald's Give In to Temptation? Available online at http://www.nytimes.com/2007/07/22/business/yourmoney/22feed.html (accessed on July 22, 2007).

Martin, Philip. 1990. Harvest of Confusion: Immigration Reform and California Agriculture. *International Migration Review* 24:69–95.

Marx, Karl. 1906. *Capital: A Critique of Political Economy.* New York: Modern Library.

Maugham, C. W. 1998. Red Meat. In *The Structure and Dynamics of New Zealand Industries,* ed. Michael Pickford and Alan Bollard, 25–52. Palmerston North, NZ: Dunmore Press.

Maurer, Bill. 2005. *Mutual Life Limited: Islamic Banking, Alternative Currencies, Lateral Reason.* Princeton, NJ: Princeton University Press.

McGee, Harold. 2004. *On Food and Cooking: The Science and Lore of the Kitchen.* New York: Scribner.

McKenna, M., M. Roche, R. Le Heron. 1999. H. J. Heinz and Global Gardens. *International Journal of the Sociology of Agriculture and Food* 8:35–51.

McMichael, Philip, ed. 1994. *The Global Restructuring of Agro-Food Systems.* Ithaca, NY: Cornell University Press.

Meat and Wool New Zealand. 2003. *The Business of New Zealand Meat.* Wellington: Country-Wide Publications.

Meta, Jack. 2009. Flap in the Face of Beef Stew. Available online at http://
  thenational.com.pg/040909/whender2.php (accessed on April 11, 2009).
Miller, Daniel. 1998. Appropriating the State on the Council Estate. *Man*
  23:353–72.
Mintz, Sidney. 1985. *Sweetness and Power: The Place of Sugar in Modern History.*
  New York: Viking Penguin.
Miyazaki, Hirokazu. 2006. Economy of Dreams: Hope in Global Capitalism
  and its Critiques. *Cultural Anthropology* 21:147–72.
Muntweiler, M., and R.M. Shelton. 2001. Survey of Nutrition and Protein Intake
  in Rural Families in Eastern Highlands Province. In *Food Security for Papua
  New Guinea*, ed. R. Michael Bourke, Matthew Allen and J.G. Salisbury,
  432–42. Canberra: Australian Centre for International Agricultural
  Research.
National Food and Nutrition Centre. 2007. *2004 National Nutrition Survey: Main
  Report.* Suva, Fiji: National Food and Nutrition Centre.
National Health Promotion Council. 2006. *Health Promotion Policy for Fiji.*
  Unpublished document, Suva, Fiji.
Neel, J.V. 1962. Diabetes Mellitus: A "Thrifty" Gene Rendered Detrimental by
  "Progress"? *American Journal of Human Genetics* 14:353–62.
New Zealand Government. 2007. Government Response to the Inquiry into
  Obesity and Type 2 Diabetes. Wellington: New Zealand Government.
New Zealand Health Committee. 2007. *Inquiry into Obesity and Type 2 Diabetes
  in New Zealand.* Wellington: New Zealand Government.
New Zealand Joint Agency Report. 2007. *Joint Report: Impact of New Zealand
  Export of Sheep Meat (Mutton and Lamb) Flaps on Obesity and Chronic Disease in
  Pacific Island Countries.* Wellington: NZ Aid, Ministry of Foreign Affairs and
  Trade, Ministry of Health.
New Zealand Ministry of Health. 2003. New Zealand Food, New Zealand
  Children. Available online at http://www.moh.govt.nz/moh.nsf/0/064234A7
  283A0478CC256DD60000AB4C/$File/nzfoodnzchildren.pdf (accessed on
  July 27, 2007).
New Zealand National Party. 2005. Official Website. Available online at http://
  www.national.org.nz/About/welcome.aspx (accessed on April 6, 2008).
O'Callaghan, Marie Louise. 1996. PNG in a Flap on Fat Food Business. *Austra-
  lian*, June 3, n.p.
Ongugo, Kindin. 2009. Not All Metabolic Diseases Caused by Lamb Flaps.
  Available online at http://thenational.com.pg/040809/letter2.php (accessed
  on April 11, 2009).
Owen, Chris. 1990. *Man with No Pigs.* Videorecording. Watertown, MA:
  Documentary Educational Resources.

Papua New Guinea Post-Courier. 2003. Viewpoint. Available online at http://www
.postcourier.com.pg/20031106/drum/htm (accessed on November 6, 2003).
———. 2005. Health Hazards in PNG. Available online at http://www.postcourier
.com.pg/20051027/news09.htm (accessed on October 27, 2005).
———. 2006. Raid on Lamb Flaps. February 16, 2006, n.p.
Parkinson, Susan. 1999. Lamb Flaps and Health. *Fiji Times*, December 17, n.p.
Pearson, Sarina. 1995. Lamb Flaps, Tourists, Pop Music and Mortuary Rites:
    Post-Colonialism and Tradition on Manam Island, Papua New Guinea. M. A.
    thesis, Department of Anthropology, University of Southern California.
Petersen, Chasa. 2005. Professor Studies Mice to Understand Obesity. Available
    online at http://www.utahstatesman.com/media/paper243/news/2005/04/
    20/Features (accessed on December 11, 2006).
Poe, Tracy. 1999. The Origins of Soul Food in Black Urban Identity: Chicago,
    1915–1974. *American Studies International* 37:4–33.
Pollan, Michael. 2006. *The Omnivore's Dilemma: A Natural History of Four Meals*.
    New York: Penguin Press.
———. 2008. *In Defense of Food: An Eater's Manifesto*. New York: Penguin Press.
Pritchard, Bill. 2005a. Implementing and Maintaining Neoliberal Agriculture
    in Australia: Part 1. *International Journal of Sociology of Agriculture and Food*
    13 (1): 1–12.
———. 2005b. Implementing and Maintaining Neoliberal Agriculture in
    Australia: Part 2. *International Journal of Sociology of Agriculture and Food*
    13 (2): 1–12.
Pritchard, Bill, and Phil McManus, eds. 2000. *Land of Discontent: The Dynamics
    of Change in Rural and Regional Australia*. Sydney: University of New South
    Wales Press.
Pryor, Ian. 1976. Nutritional Problems in Pacific Islanders. Unpublished
    transcript of the Muriel Bell Memorial Lecture, Wellington, New Zealand.
Rappaport, Roy. 1968. *Pigs for the Ancestors: Ritual and the Ecology of a New
    Guinea People*. New Haven, CT: Yale University Press.
Reid, Roddy. 2005. *Globalizing Tobacco Control: Anti-Smoking Campaigns in
    California, France, and Japan*. Bloomington: University of Indiana Press.
Reuters. 2006. Kenya Offended at Dog Food Aid Offer. Available online at http://
    today.reuters.com/misc/PrinterFriendlyPopup.aspx?type+oddlyEnoughNews
    &storyID (accessed February 8, 2006).
Rex. 2005. Two Anthropologists, One Piece of Meat. Available online at http://
    savageminds.org/2005/06/20/two-anthropologists-one-piece-of-meat
    (accessed on March 11, 2006).
Richter, Richard. 1985. *Hungry for Profit*. Videorecording. Ho-Ho-Kus, NJ: New
    Day Films.

Rose, Lisa. 2001. Meat and Early Human Diet: Insights from Neotropical Primate Studies. In *Meat-Eating and Human Evolution*, ed. Craig Stanford and Henry Bunn, 141–78. Oxford: Oxford University Press.

Sahlins, Marshall. 1985. *Islands of History*. Chicago: University of Chicago Press.

———. 1992. The Economics of Develop-Man in the Pacific. *Res* 21:13–25.

Sakaue, Motoyoshi, Yoko Fuke, Toshie Katsuyama, Masato Kawabat, and Hiroshi Taniguchi. 2003. Austronesian-Speaking People in Papua New Guinea Have Susceptibility to Obesity and Type 2 Diabetes. *Diabetes Care*. Available online at http://care.diabetesjournals.org/cgi/content/full/26/3/955-a (accessed on June 15, 2008).

Saweri, Wila. 2001. The Rocky Road from Roots to Rice: A Review of the Changing Food and Nutrition Situation in Papua New Guinea. *Papua New Guinea Medical Journal* 44:51–163.

Schieffelin, Edward. 1976. *The Sorrow of the Lonely and the Burning of the Dancers*. New York: St. Martin's Press.

Schlosser, Eric. 2002. *Fast Food Nation: The Dark Side of the All-American Meal*. New York: Perennial

Schultz, Jimaima, Gade Waqa, Marita McCabe, Lina Ricciardelli, and Helen Mavoa. 2006. *Report on Interviews with Indigenous Fijian and IndoFijian Youth: Sociocultural Studies in the Healthy Youth Healthy Community Project*. Unpublished Report, OPIC Project, Fiji School of Medicine and Deakin University School of Psychology, Suva and Melbourne.

Scragg, Robert. 2006. Developing and Evaluating *Obesity* Prevention In Communities: The OPIC Study. Powerpoint presentation, Faculty of Medical and Health Sciences, University of Auckland.

Seneviratne, Asoka. 2001. Fat: The Good, The Bad, The Ugly. *Reporter*, October 26.

Simmons, David, and Justine Mesui. 1999. Decisional Balance and State of Change in Relation to Weight Loss, Exercise and Dietary Fat Reduction among Pacific Island People. *Asia Pacific Journal of Clinical Nutrition* 8:39–45.

Sims, Laura. 1998. *The Politics of Fat: Food and Nutrition Policy in America*. Armonk, NY: M. E. Sharpe.

Sinclair, Upton. 2001. *The Jungle*. New York: Signet. (Orig. pub. 1906.)

Slatter, Claire. 2003. Will Trade Liberalisation Lead to the Eradication or the Exacerbation of Poverty? Paper presented to the Trade Forum, St. John's Church, Wellington, New Zealand, February 21.

Smil, Vaclav. 2002. Eating Meat: Evolution, Patterns, and Consequences. *Population and Development Review* 28: 599–639.

Sobal, Jeffery. 1999. Food System, Globalization, Eating Transformations, and Nutrition Transitions. In *Food in Global History*, ed. Raymond Grew, 171–93. Boulder, CO: Westview Press.

South Pacific Commission. 2005. Vision and Mission. Available online at http://www.spc.int/corp/index.php?option = com_content&task = view&id = 22& Itemid = 73 (accessed on October 30, 2006).

South Pacific Consumer Protection Programme. 1997. *What Is the Problem with Mutton Flaps?* Unpublished report, Wainuiomata, New Zealand.

Speth, John, and Katherine Spielmann. 1983. Energy Source, Protein Metabolism, and Hunter-Gatherer Subsistence Strategies. *Journal of Anthropological Archaeology* 2:1–31.

Speth, John, and Eitan Tchernov. 2001. Neandertal Hunting and Meat-Processing in the Near East: Evidence from Kebara Cave (Israel). In *Meat-Eating and Human Evolution*, ed. Craig Stanford and Henry Bunn, 52–72. Oxford: Oxford University Press.

Spurlock, Morgan. 2004. *Super Size Me.* Videorecording. New York: Hart Sharp Video.

Stanford, Craig. 2001. A Comparison of Social Meat-Foraging by Chimpanzee and Human Foragers. In *Meat-Eating and Human Evolution*, ed. Craig Stanford and Henry Bunn, 122–40. Oxford: Oxford University Press.

Striffler, Steve. 2005. *Chicken: The Dangerous Transformation of America's Favorite Food*. New Haven, CT: Yale University Press.

Stull, Donald, and Michael Broadway. 2004. *Slaughterhouse Blues: The Meat and Poultry Industry in North America*. Belmont, CA: Wadsworth.

Sullivan, Nancy, Thomas Warr, Joseph Rainbubu, Jennifer Kunoko, Francis Akauna, Moses Angasa, and Yunus Wenda. 2003. *Tinpis Maror: A Social Impact Study of the Proposed R. D. Tuna Cannery at Vidar Wharf, Madang*. Unpublished report. Available online at http://www.nancysullivan.org/companyreports.htm.

Swinburn, Boyd. 2004. Proposal to Introduce a Bill to Restrict the Availability of Imported Fatty Meats on the Tongan Marketplace. Unpublished draft, Cabinet Briefing Paper.

Taufa, Tkutau, and Amos Benjamin. 2001. Diabetes: The By-Product of Westernization in Papua New Guinea. *Papua New Guinea Medical Journal* 44:108–110.

Templeton, Sarah-Kate. 2008. Burger Bars Face Ban Near Playgrounds. Available online at http://Timesonline.co.uk/tol/news/uk/health/articles3216727.ece (accessed on April 12, 2009).

Temu, Puka. 1991. Adult Medicine and the New Killer Diseases in Papua New Guinea. *Papua New Guinea Medical Journal* 34:1–5.

Temu, Puka, and Wila Saweri. 2001. Nutrition in Transition. In *Food Security for Papua New Guinea*, ed. R. Michael Bourke, Matthew Allen and J. G. Salisbury, 395–406. Canberra: Australian Centre for International Agricultural Research.

Texas Association for School Nutrition. 2005. Legislative Update. Available online at http://www.tsfsa.org/doc.asp?id = 229&archive = t (accessed on January 4, 2008).

Thomas, Nicholas. 1991. *Entangled Objects: Exchange, Material Culture, and Colonialism in the Pacific.* Cambridge, MA: Harvard University Press.

Trostle, James. 2005. *Epidemiology and Culture.* Cambridge: Cambridge University Press.

Trostle, James, and Johannes Sommerfeld. 1996. Medical Anthropology and Epidemiology. *Annual Review of Anthropology* 25:253–74.

Ufkes, Frances. 1998. Building a Better Pig: Fat Profits in Lean Meat. In *Animal Geographies: Place, Politics, and Identity in the Nature-Culture Borderlands,* ed. Jennifer Wolch and Jody Emel, 241–55. London: Verso.

Vatucawaqa, Penina. 2002. The Ubiquitous Noodles. In *Determinants of Food Choice in Fiji,* ed. Kate Owen. Canberra: Australian Centre for International Agricultural Research.

Vatucawaqa, Penina, and Josephine Chand. 2002. Understanding Protein Choices in Fiji. In *Determinants of Food Choice in Fiji,* ed. Kate Owen. Canberra: Australian Centre for International Agricultural Research.

Vatucawaqa, Penina, and Kate Owen. 2002. Patterns of Food Consumption for Fijians. In *Determinants of Food Choice in Fiji,* ed. Kate Owen. Canberra: Australian Centre for International Agricultural Research.

Vialles, Noëlie. 1994. *Animal to Edible.* Cambridge: Cambridge University Press.

Vinit, Thomas. 2009. Efforts to Ban Lamb Flaps. Available online at http://thenational.com.pg/040609/letter1.php (accessed on April 11, 2009).

Walsh, Rebecca, and Francesca Mold. 2003. NZ PM Gives Tuvalu Patient a Lifeline. Available online at http://www.tuvaluislands.com/news/archived/2003/2003–05–13a.htm (accessed on May 1, 2004).

Watson, James. 1997. *Golden Arches East: McDonald's in East Asia.* Stanford, CA: Stanford University Press.

West, Paige. n.d. *From Modern Production to Imagined Primitive: Tracking the Commodity Ecumene for Papua New Guinean Coffee.* Unpublished book manuscript.

Willett, Walter. 2001. *Eat, Drink and Be Healthy: The Harvard Medical School Guide to Healthy Eating.* New York: Free Press.

World Health Organization. 2007. A Guide to Statistical Information at WHO. Available online at http://www.who.int/whosis/en/index.html (accessed on January 17, 2008).

Wrangham, Richard, James Holland Jones, Greg Laden, David Pilbeam, and NancyLou Conklin-Brittain. 1999. The Raw and the Stolen. *Current Anthropology* 40: 567–94.

Wratten, Adam. 2002. Toilet-Time Penalty Sparks Dispute Meat Union Says: It Stinks. Available online at http://www.amieu.asn.au/printout.php?recid = 43 (accessed on May 6, 2007).

Yamamoto, Atsuko. n.d. Shall We Diet. Translation of an article that appeared in *UNO* magazine and was sent to Robert Hughes in 1997.

Zaloom, Caitlin. 2003. Ambiguous Numbers: Trading Technologies and Interpretations in Financial Markets. *American Ethnologist* 30:258–72.

———. 2004. The Productive Life of Risk. *Cultural Anthropology* 19:365–91.

Index

political economy of, 145; obesity and
diabetes in, 23, 88; quota recommended
on fatty meats in, 144–46; regulatory
experimentation needed in, 164; weight
loss tales from, 150–52
totems, flaps as, 25, 30, 49, 116, 161
tuna, 3, 87, 110
Tupou IV (King of Tonga), 50, 150–51, 153,
190n20, 191n21
turkey tails, 146–47, 189n53
Twinkies, 168n8
Twisties, 3

under-nutrition, in Papua New Guinea,
89–90
United Kingdom, 31, 160

United States: beef intestines from, 179n13;
chicken from, 59; meat grading in,
172n42; meat in 1800s diet in, 20; politics
of personal choice in, 153–56, 158, 164;
as primary market for beef brisket, 73;
slaughterhouses in, 37, 38; turkey tails
from, 146

value, labor, 27

Waga, Gade, 135–36
Wamira, 171n20
Wari, 17, 171n22
Wewak, Papua New Guinea, 78–80
Willett, Walter, 45
World Trade Organization, 117, 145

Text:	10/14 Palatino
Display:	Univers Condensed Light, Bauer Bodoni
Compositor:	Binghamton Valley Composition, LLC
Indexer:	Andrew Christenson
Printer and binder:	Maple-Vail Book Manufacturing Group